T5-CCW-786

PLACE IN RETURN BOX to remove this checkout from your record.
TO AVOID FINES return on or before date due.
MAY BE RECALLED with earlier due date if requested.

DATE DUE	DATE DUE	DATE DUE
JAN 30 07 2 2002		
DEC 11 02 2003		
MAY 05 02 4 2005		
OCT 2 9 0 2005		
MAY 1 5 2006		
0 5 0 1 0 6		
NOV 12 8 2007 0 7		

11/00 c:/CIRC/DateDue.p65-p.14

ABORTION

Changing Views and Practice

FEB '73

Seminars in Psychiatry

ABORTION;
Changing Views and Practice

R. BRUCE SLOANE, M.D., *Editor*

GRUNE & STRATTON **New York and London**

A Note From the Publisher

This book is reprinted in large part from the August 1970 issue (Vol. 2, No. 3) of *Seminars in Psychiatry*, published by Henry M. Stratton, Inc., 757 Third Avenue, New York, N.Y. 10017. It contains, in addition, updated material on the New York State successes and problems in dealing with the most liberal abortion law in this country.

Seminars in Psychiatry is a quarterly journal, Milton Greenblatt, M.D., Editor-in-Chief, Ernest Hartmann, M.D., Associate Editor. It is *topical* in nature; that is, each issue deals with a single topic of major importance to today's understanding and clinical practice of psychiatry, with invited experts contributing articles, based on their own experience, which review that topic from various viewpoints. Each issue is thus, in effect, a soft-cover monograph—current, authoritative, stimulating and usable. The journal has published:

VOLUME 1, 1969

No. 1 (Feb.): Adolescence, *Topic Editor, Ernest Hartmann, M.D.*
No. 2 (May): The Amphetamines in Psychiatry, *Topic Editor, Jonathan O. Cole, M.D.*
No. 3 (Aug.): Learning Disabilities: Integrity and Usefulness as Diagnostic and Treatment Concepts, *Topic Editor, Burton Blatt, Ed.D.*
No. 4 (Nov.): Brief Psychiatric Treatment, *Topic Editor, Seymour Fisher, Ph.D.*

VOLUME 2, 1970

No. 1 (Feb.): Behavior Genetics, *Topic Editor, Stanley Walzer, M.D.*
No. 2 (May): Psychiatric Education for the Seventies, *Topic Editor, Jack R. Ewalt, M.D.*
No. 3 (Aug.): Psychiatric Aspects of Abortion, *Topic Editor, R. Bruce Sloane, M.D.*
No. 4 (Nov.): Natural History of Mental Illness: 10–50-Year Follow-up Studies, *Topic Editor, George E. Vaillant, M.D.*

Information about subscribing or purchasing individual copies may be obtained from Henry M. Stratton, Inc., Subscription Department, 757 Third Avenue, New York, N.Y. 10017.

Library of Congress Catalog Card Number 72-150000
International Standard Book Number 0-8089-0683-6

Printed in the United States of America (G-B)

Contents

CONTRIBUTORS vii

INTRODUCTION .... R. Bruce Sloane 1

Attitudes

ABORTION DOGMAS NEEDING RESEARCH SCRUTINY .... Edward Pohlman 10

TO WHOM DOES THE CHILD BELONG?
     Alan A. Stone, Milton Greenblatt, Jack Ewalt and William Curran 21

LEGAL ASPECTS OF ABORTION .... Samuel Polsky 36

ABORTION: THE CATHOLIC VIEWPOINT .... Frank J. Ayd, Jr. 48

ABORTION: THE MENTAL HEALTH CONSEQUENCES OF UNWANTEDNESS
                                  Mildred B. Beck 53

THE GYNECOLOGIST AND "THERAPEUTIC" ABORTION: THE CHANGING TIMES
            Russell Ramon de Alvarez and Martin B. Wingate 65

Reviews and Studies

PSYCHOLOGICAL AND EMOTIONAL INDICATIONS FOR
    THERAPEUTIC ABORTION .... Nathan M. Simon 73

FETAL "INDICATIONS" FOR TERMINATION OF PREGNANCY ... Henry L. Nadler 92

ABORTION ATTITUDES OF POVERTY-LEVEL BLACKS
     Clark E. Vincent, C. Allen Haney and Carl M. Cochrane 99

SOCIOECONOMIC ASPECTS OF ABORTION .... David Goldberg 108

THERAPEUTIC ABORTION IN GREAT BRITAIN .... D. A. Pond 126

AGE, MARRIAGE, PERSONALITY AND DISTRESS: A STUDY OF PERSONALITY
    FACTORS IN WOMEN REFERRED FOR THERAPEUTIC ABORTION
                                Peter C. Olley 131

ABORTION OR NO? WHAT DECIDES? AN INQUIRY BY QUESTIONNAIRE INTO THE
    ATTITUDES OF GYNECOLOGISTS AND PSYCHIATRISTS IN ABERDEEN
                        C. McCance and P. F. McCance 142

THE COLORADO REPORT .... Abraham Heller and H. G. Whittington 151

ABORTION ON REQUEST: ITS CONSEQUENCES FOR POPULATION TRENDS
    AND PUBLIC HEALTH .... Christopher Tietze 165

THE CHANGING PRACTICE OF ABORTION
              R. Bruce Sloane and Diana F. Horvitz 172

INDEX 181

Contributors

Frank J. Ayd, Jr., M.D., Editor, *The Medical-Moral Newsletter*, Baltimore, Md.

Mildred B. Beck, M.S.W., Acting Chief, Office of Information and Education, National Center for Family Planning Services, Rockville, Md.

Carl M. Cochrane, Ph.D., Professor of Psychology, Behavioral Sciences Center, The Bowman Gray School of Medicine, Wake Forest University, Winston-Salem, N.C.

William Curran, L.L.M., Sc.M., Frances Glessner Lee Professor of Legal Medicine, Harvard University School of Public Health, Cambridge, Mass.

Russell Ramon de Alvarez, M.D., Professor and Chairman Emeritus, Department of Obstetrics and Gynecology, Temple University School of Medicine, Temple University Health Sciences Center, Philadelphia, Pa.

Jack Ewalt, M.D., Bullard Professor of Psychiatry, Harvard Medical School, Cambridge, Mass.; Superintendent, Massachusetts Mental Health Center, Boston, Mass.

David Goldberg, M.A., M.R.C.P., D.P.M., Senior Lecturer in Psychiatry, Manchester University, Manchester, England.

Milton Greenblatt, M.D., Commissioner of Mental Health, Commonwealth of Massachusetts; Professor of Psychiatry, Tufts University School of Medicine, Medford, Mass.

C. Allen Haney, Ph.D., Assistant Professor of Sociology, Behavioral Sciences Center, The Bowman Gray School of Medicine, Wake Forest University, Winston-Salem, N.C.

Abraham Heller, M.D., Assistant Director, Division of Psychiatric Services, City and County of Denver, Denver, Colo.

Diana F. Horvitz, B.A., Research Assistant, Department of Psychiatry, Temple University School of Medicine, Temple University Health Sciences Center, Philadelphia, Pa.

C. McCance, M.A., M.B., M.R.C.P., Consultant Psychiatrist, Department of Mental Health, Northeastern Region of Scotland; Department of Mental Health Research Unit, University of Aberdeen, Scotland.

P. F. McCance, M.R.C.S., L.R.C.P., M.B., B.S., Research Assistant, Department of Mental Health, Northeastern Region of Scotland.

Henry L. Nadler, M.D., Given Research Professor of Pediatrics, Department of Pediatrics, Northwestern University Medical School; Head of the Division of Genetics, Children's Memorial Hospital, Chicago, Ill.

Peter C. Olley, M.B., Ch.B., B.Sc., Dip. Psych. (Ed.), Lecturer in Mental Health, Mental Health Research Unit, University of Aberdeen, Aberdeen, Scotland.

Edward Pohlman, Ph.D., Professor of Educational and Counseling Psychology, University of the Pacific, Stockton, Calif.

Samuel Polsky, LL.B., Ph.D., Professor of Law and Psychiatry, Temple University School of Law, Philadelphia, Pa.

D. A. Pond, M.D., F.R.C.P., D.P.M., Professor of Psychiatry, The London Medical College, University of London, London, England.

Nathan M. Simon, M.D., Director, Department of Psychiatry, The Jewish Hospital, St. Louis, Mo.

R. Bruce Sloane, M.D., Professor and Chairman, Department of Psychiatry, Temple University School of Medicine, Temple University Health Sciences Center, Philadelphia, Pa.

Alan A. Stone, M.D., Associate Professor of Psychiatry, Harvard Medical School; Lecturer in Law, Harvard Law School, Cambridge, Mass.

Christopher Tietze, M.D., Associate Director, Bio-Medical Division, The Population Council, New York, N.Y.

Clarke E. Vincent, Ph.D., Director, Behavioral Sciences Center, The Bowman Gray School of Medicine, Wake Forest University, Winston-Salem, N.C.

H. G. Whittington, M.D., Director, Division of Psychiatric Services, City and County of Denver, Denver Colo.

Martin B. Wingate, M.D., Professor, Department of Obstetrics and Gynecology, Temple University Health Sciences Center, Philadelphia, Pa.

Introduction

A N APPROPRIATE SUBTITLE for this issue, inspired by a recent book on sex, might be: "Things You Always Knew About Abortion But Were Wrong." Dogma of both the right and left is exposed in the clear daylight of Pohlman's writing. The topic has been so deeply buried in beliefs and misbelief that the facts were mostly unobtainable and are still hard to come by. However, just as the sixties seemed to be an uncovering decade revealing both the female form and sexual habits, it now seems appropriate that the seventies should reveal what has been called the most fundamental and least understood area of human behavior, namely the role of abortion in the total reproductive process.[2]

The Voice of Women

Although traditionally the attitudes of men shaped both the law and practice of abortion, women's views are becoming increasingly heard. Betty Friedan, a founder of the National Organization for Women, blazed the trail of the modern feminist movement eight years ago when she indicted the traditional image of the American housewife in *The Feminine Mystique*. She now expresses herself forcibly on the issue of abortion.

> In the whole unfinished sexual revolution in America—the revolution of American women toward full participation in society—there is no freedom, no equality, no full human dignity and personhood possible for women until they assert and demand control over their own bodies and their own reproductive process. To enable all women, not just the exceptional few, to move in society, we must accept as a fact of life, a temporary fact of most women's life today, that women do give birth to children. But it is left to all women to challenge the idea that it is their primary role to bear and rear children. There is only one voice that needs to be heard on the question of whether a woman will or will not bear a child and that is the voice of the woman herself. The right to have an abortion is a matter of individual conscience and conscious choice for the woman concerned.[4]

Anne Vaillant[15] points to laws that decree that a wife may be forced against her will to have intercourse with her husband but that she may not procure an abortion without masculine consent. In this way two central expressions of female sexuality, pregnancy and birth, are removed from her control. In contrast man is assured of full control of his own male sexuality. She urges women to speak up and men to listen.

Alice Rossi,[14] perhaps more tellingly, points to the acceptance of the nurtu-

1

rant maternal female role by women themselves. Only by giving birth to children can they gain approval. Maternity, she says, cannot continue to be an exclusive goal of women for this encourages the view that the more children the better, as well as the view that no marriage is complete without a child. Praise and social approval of women with large numbers of children are no longer appropriate to a crowded urban society. This applies to economically affluent women as well as to poor women, to American women as well as to Latin-American women, to white women as well as to black women. She considers that the major problem is the reduction in the rate of "wanted" pregnancies. In the United States in 1966, an average of 3.4 children was considered ideal by white women aged 21 and older. In her own research, college graduates had the desired family size, namely 3.2 and 38 per cent of them desired four children or more.

The basic motivation for having children must be changed, she urges, and such an approach must necessarily involve changes in the structure of the family and sexual mores. There must be opportunities for legitimate alternative satisfaction apart from the family role. In practice she considers that legal change to permit women to abort unwanted pregnancies would seem to be the easiest way to cope with the population problem. It would involve the removal of barriers women do not want rather than the more difficult task of changing deep-lying motivations.

Mildred Beck's cri de coeur is not unexpectedly directed in another direction. As a social worker she deplores laws which condemn many an unborn child to the hazards of an unwanted life at the hands of a feckless mother.

The Law

If the law is supreme then it should be recognized as man-made and, as Polsky points out, shaped much by religious attitudes. The law in fact recognizes the fetus as a special aggregation of cells with a potential for independent life and in this way protects the rights of the unborn child. Legal rights such as the right to inherit, the right to sue, the right not to be harmed by drugs, and the right to bring a tort action, can, in fact, be extended to say that the fetus has a right to a life of its own, and this argument is debated by Curran and Stone in their discussion of the GAP report. Neither they nor Polsky favor the American Law Institute recommendations. Polsky considers that these recommendations inject another brand of morality into the situation in terms of what social consequences are adverse enough to justify an abortion. In fact they defer such matters to medical judgment and in introducing the concept of the physician's good faith, the law would delegate special responsibility to him. Such a situation has, of course, existed for many years in Scotland and seems to have operated quite favorably.

MacGillivray who, with his colleagues, has produced one of the finest studies extant[10] says that termination of pregnancy in Aberdeen was often performed even though there was no immediate risk to the life of the mother. The abortion rate in Scotland, 2.4 per thousand women aged 15-44, has remained the same as the rate in National Health Service hospitals in England

and Wales since the passing of the new Act. In Aberdeen, however, while therapeutic abortion for married women has remained the same over the last decade, there has been a steep rise in terminations of pregnancy in single women and illegitimate pregnancies. The latter terminations have increased some fourteen-fold, and in 1968 one-third of all illegitimate pregnancies were so ended. This Aberdeen experience would seem to illustrate how even when a law is liberally interpreted it still greatly influences behavior. Change in the law, in fact, allows much more freedom of choice and for the first time some succor for the illegitimately pregnant young girl.

The GAP report "The Right to Abortion: A Psychiatric View"[13] recommends that abortion, when performed by a licensed physician, should be entirely removed from the domain of criminal law. Laws as currently enforced, they say, impose enormous hardship on the unwilling mother. The writers believe that a woman should have the right to abort or not just as she has the right to marry or not.{"There can be nothing more destructive to a child's spirit than being unwanted and there are few things more destructive to a woman's spirit than being forced without love or need into motherhood." }

In their discussion "To Whom does the Child Belong?" our contributors Stone, Greenblatt, Ewalt and Curran spiritedly debate this issue. Curran, in particular, criticizes the "rights of the woman." He points out that these are not the same as the "right to marry"; they are not the same as the "right to vote." Certainly the *mother* has no greater right to force a doctor to terminate her pregnancy than she has to persuade him to remove any other part of her body. The *father* has few rights. He cannot insist that pregnancy with his child go to term. Still less, as Stone points out, can he force his wife to bring his child up properly. At present this responsibility falls to the very woman who did not want the child. This leads Stone to the conclusion that the least tragic way out of the dilemma is for the mother to have the say. Polsky disagrees, in part, with this notion. He maintains that the responsibility for the fetus belongs to the mother only until viability, a view in accord with the recently passed law of New York State.

Religion

The most clear and concise religious position is that of the Catholics and this is succinctly stated by Ayd. Most would respect his viewpoint. However, Catholics do not need the law to support their moral principles, and such religious beliefs should not be imposed by law on those who do not hold them. "There remains the moral issue of abortion as murder . . . we suggest that those who believe that abortion is murder need not avail themselves of it. On the other hand we do not believe that such conviction should limit the free- dom of those not bound by identical religious conviction. . ."[13]

Milhaven[11] reaches beyond conservative Catholic rhetoric when he says that the laws of the nation should treat men who favor abortion as a mature segment of a pluralistic society. The law should not prohibit their carrying out their basic moral conviction.

In practice, whatever the view of their church, Catholic women seek abortion as much as their non-Catholic sisters.[5,7]

The Decision

Few, except the militant feminists, agree that the decision should rest only with the woman. If she is to be advised by a physician hopefully he (or she) should be as open-minded as possible. They seldom have been in the past.

Goldberg underlines that when social events are used to justify abortion this only reveals what individual doctors have done and not what they ought to have done or what is desirable. Such idiosyncratic behavior may lead a physician to reject the young, unmarried woman who most needs the abortion. McCance and McCance illustrate the highly individual decisions of doctors. However, the physician seldom advised abortion if the woman seemed in two minds about it. If anxiety, depression, or social adversity were present, the abortion was usually granted. Interestingly enough, single women were not discriminated against nor did hints of suicide influence the decision.

Less than one-third of the patients were referred to psychiatrists. Where both psychiatrists and gynecologists saw the same patient their opinions were very similar. These findings suggest that routine psychiatric referrals are both unnecessary and in terms of the delay they cause probably harmful. They also lend substance to Pohlman's plea for better validation of assessment procedures.

Goldberg joins Pohlman in concluding that psychiatrists do not have a monopoly on human understanding. Psychiatrists are certainly much less consulted in Aberdeen or Britain in general and to require them for routine applications undoubtedly slows the process of termination and adds to its risk. Until such time as early safe abortifacients are introduced (and if the present promise of prostglandin is fulfilled,[6] this is just around the corner), women in the U.S.A. will probably have to rely on gynecologists to abort them. To this task they bring their own bias as DeAlvarez and Wingate illustrate in pointing to the dilemma of the gynecologist trained to save life, committed in abortion to its destruction. Their understandably antithetical attitudes have been mirrored in both Colorado and Britain. Implicitly they ask who should carry out society's dirty work. Many persons advocating abortion, they say, might change their mind if they were present during the destruction of the fetus, and still more if they were called upon to do the task themselves. However, if society demands a service somebody should perform it. Pohlman appropriately raises the anomoly of nonobstetricians being allowed to handle normal deliveries while they are prohibited from performing the far safer therapeutic abortion. The abortion pill may well rescue us from this debate.

The GAP report suggests that the physician who is asked to perform the abortion should be expected to exercise medical judgment as he would in the case of elective surgery. The writers particularly emphasize the importance of the physician exploring with the pregnant woman the basis of her motivation in the decision to abort. They do not believe that psychiatric consultation should necessarily be routine and most would agree.

However, their recommendation somewhat minimizes the intense emotions aroused by abortion which seldom obtain in other areas of elective surgery.

Stone wisely doubts medical omniscience and, just as in other areas of elective surgery, it is likely that the determined woman will eventually get her wish whatever her "rights" may be.

Who Gets an Abortion

Goldberg points out that the very woman whom society might agree should desirably receive an abortion, especially the poor, married or single are the ones most denied it under restricted laws. Even when the law is liberalized the poor are slow to take advantage of it.

This is illustrated in the findings of Aitken-Swan[1] which revealed that in Aberdeen, in the years 1963-1965, only 3 per cent of the single women who were unskilled manual workers having a baby or an abortion received a therapeutic abortion, compared with 63 per cent of the professional group. However, if they were referred for termination, as many of these working class girls (60 per cent) were granted it as were the professional ones. Aitken-Swan raised the question whether such girls did not ask their physicians for an abortion or did ask him but were more easily put off by a negative attitude or whether the girl and her parents were more tolerant of an illegitimate pregnancy and ready to accept the baby into the family.

Heller and Whittington say that different practices of the past were dependent on the social status of the single pregnant girl. The middle and upper class one often went to the home for unwed mothers and the baby was ultimately given up for adoption. The lower class girl, especially if she were poor, black and/or Spanish, usually retained her baby which was often looked after by her mother. Neither of these practices seem to have been significantly affected by the greater availability of therapeutic abortions in Colorado. Poor people, of course, may just be slow in finding out about a new service. Moreover, if doctors really were swayed by bad social conditions in making their recommendations for termination then it would be reasonable, says Goldberg, to expect that the socioeconomic status of those accepted would be worse than for those refused. This, he points out, is not true of either the Swedish or Colorado data (nor of the Aberdonian).

Diggory[2] suggests that the "establishment" girl in Britain probably obtained a private abortion and undoubtedly the same obtained in this country.

Olley draws a poignant picture of the single girl who applies for abortion in Aberdeen. She is an intelligent but impulsive isolated girl who has interpersonal difficulties and who, in spite of her self-doubt, is often stubborn and assertive. He uses the term "accident prone" to describe her, but the casualness with which three-quarters of them had never taken any precautions against conception might argue for a certain determinism in their behavior. The married woman was a somewhat insecure, serious, and anxious woman burdened down with cares. Olley concluded that illegitimate pregnancy was often predisposed to by the woman's personality and not due to unfortunate circumstances, a modest conclusion few clinicians would disagree with.

Who Should Get an Abortion?

Simon stresses the key issue of "unwantedness." From his own studies and an extensive review of the literature he concludes that any woman with a determined desire to end her pregnancy should have an abortion and does well following this. He somewhat sharply draws attention to the ridiculous Cartesian duality of "medical" and "psychological" indications. He underlines that suicide and psychosis are not as isolated occurrences as many claim but stigmatize those who seek only such coarse indices of psychological stress.

Emotional symptoms following abortion are not common and seldom new in the life of the woman experiencing them. They may well have occurred even had the woman borne her child to term. Moreover, as Pohlman points out, 'guilt' following abortion is likely to be tempered by the prevailing social climate and lessened by its degree of liberalness.

Simon's evidence points overwhelmingly to the view that as far as the *woman's* welfare and health is concerned anyone who unambivalently wants an abortion should be granted one.

The Fetus

Nadler illustrates clearly how even with advances of scientific knowledge and techniques such as intrauterine diagnosis, the degree of risk and of malformation will often remain unknown. Laws cannot define such risks but where termination for fetal conditions is legal the parents might make their own individual decision aided by the advice of their physician. This will allow them to exercise their own morality.

The Unwanted Child

Mildred Beck, in her description of the evils of unwantedness, perhaps diminishes the force of her argument by overgeneralizing it, from murderers through suiciders to schizophrenics. It seems unlikely that in the multiple etiology of schizophrenia, unwantedness looms large. Although she pleads for a definition of the term, Pohlman in his excellent book *The Psychology of Birth Planning*[12] suggests that the concept is so ambiguous that research based upon it should be abandoned. Admitting to an unwanted conception clearly requires frankness of the woman, he says. It may be that the correlate of this verbal behavior, namely frankness, would be at least partly responsible for any differences noted in reported angry feelings toward the child, harsh punishments, emotional upsets and so on. Instead, he recommends looking into criteria such as family size (a large family is more likely to have a larger number of unwanted pregnancies) timing of births in relationship to the mother's age and when she was married, the sex composition of the family, whether conception and birth occur out of wedlock, and other such more definable incidents.

He himself began his work with the high hope that he would find convincing research data that unwanted conceptions tended to have undesirable effects for parents and children. However, his extensive review of the literature unearthed very little evidence of this sort and what evidence there was, with the exception that induced abortion was much more likely after unwanted conception, was not very convincing. Nevertheless he pointed to the abundant expert opinion summed up by Finch:[3]

> Mental health workers would agree that being unplanned and especially unwanted is usually detrimental to the child's emotional development and perhaps also to that of his siblings. The conclusion is reached primarily from clinical experience and there is no available statistical study with adequate controls which would prove the point. Such data would be difficult to obtain for a variety of reasons but should be sought.

In conclusion, Pohlman doubts whether research on the effects of unwanted conception would have great practical value in advancing the cause of birth planning. The threat of over-population, he feels, is likely to be a far more powerful incentive to influence people to promote such planning. Moreover, he continues, many people seem to be convinced that unwanted births have undesirable effects, and the lack of research does not diminish the extent of their feelings nor would the extent of their feelings be increased much by a clear research report. Advocates of the child are still all too scarce and Mildred Beck, a stout one, would say 'Amen'!

What Are the Consequences of Changing the Law?

If the new law is liberal and in Britain, its results seem only to be good: if it is not so liberal, and in Colorado, the results seem not so good. Clearly, culture may be as important a determinant of the results as are the legal statutes.

Pond suggests that the fact that gynecologists are solidly against abortion on demand (although paradoxically in favor of sterilization) may have contributed to the growth of private abortion clinics. However most of the controversy around these seems more moral than medical. No one claims that they are harming the health of women. Rather, critics are concerned either with the cupidity of their operators or with the wages of sin which they feel should not be cashed so readily. As Diggory and his colleagues point out, only 7 per cent of abortions have been done on foreigners (many of them in any case temporarily resident in England) ridiculing the jibes that London had become the abortion capitol of the world.[2]

An argument frequently raised is that pressure of therapeutic abortions squeezes out the treatment of more needed and "desirable" obstetrical and gynecological conditions. This does not seem to have been borne out in Britain. Indeed, somewhat mischievously, Pohlman points out that if obstetricians spent more time doing therapeutic abortions they would have less need for the time consuming business of delivering babies. However, at the Denver General Hospital, as Heller and Whittington illustrate, an unfair share of the state's abortion practice may well produce pressure on a service, accentuating inimical attitudes to the procedure.

Heller and Whittington urge that psychiatry should proselytize changing attitudes to the medical profession and society. In Britain mere change of the law seems to be changing medical attitudes. Before the Act, Diggory points out, few general practitioners referred their patients to National Health Service gynecologists for termination unless the grounds were exceptional.

Now, although the reason, namely to protect the physical or mental health of the pregnant woman, is little altered from previously, the referral is made and the woman comes face to face with the gynecologist. This forces him to appreciate something of the extent of the despair and distress associated with the unwanted pregnancy and his reaction has been largely humane as expressed by the granting of abortion on an increasing scale. Bodies such as the Royal College of Obstetricians and Gynecologists are now taking a sincere if belated interest in contraception and sterilization.

Forty per cent of all abortions done since the Act were on single women. Preliminary birth returns for the first half of 1969 revealed a slowing down in the illegitimacy rate which had been rising steeply since 1958 (an estimated 34,000 compared with 69,806 in 1968). Some 20,000 terminations were carried out on the unmarried girls in the first year of the Act.

In 1969 there were in England and Wales 6.8 legal abortions per 100 live births, compared with the Swedish figures of 10, the Hungarian of 135.6, and the Japanese of 38.7. The Act has worked well in placing the decision in the hands of doctors and there has been minimal delay in seeking abortion and its performance which contrasts to the Scandinavian tribunal procedure (and Colorado) where long delays have both discouraged women from using legal abortion and resulted in the terminations being performed later and therefore less safely.

Heller and Whittington, from their experience at the Denver General Hospital, point out that even though the numbers of therapeutic abortions increased eighteenfold over those done under the old law, the rate of therapeutic abortion compared to live births has scarcely moved out of range of the national average estimated years ago and was nowhere near that of the Scandinavian and Eastern European countries or Japan. They estimate that medical abortions in Colorado are now probably a mere 10 per cent of all induced abortions and are probably for the first time beginning to make a significant inroad into nonmedical abortion practice. Some three-fifths of all applicants were single girls, half of whom were unemancipated teenagers. The poor, especially if Indian, Spanish-American or black, remain sparsely represented.

Hospitals and their staffs in Colorado seem to be embarrassed by legal, although still restricted, abortion. They often set up boards and regulations which frustrate even the limited objectives of the new bill.[8] State representative Richard Lamm, chief sponsor of Colorado's reform law, recently summarized the feelings of many critics by saying that the reform just was not good enough. "We tried to change a cruel, outmoded, inhuman law—and what we got was a cruel, outmoded, inhuman law," he said. "We still force women either to have a baby or to have an illegal abortion."[9]

On the positive side, Heller and Whittington showed that emotional rejection of the abortion patients by the obstetrical team at the Denver General Hospital could be alleviated by a full time psychiatric nurse and inservice training. Moreover, although 90 per cent of those granted abortion qualified on the grounds of quite serious impairment of mental health, the patient with a history of prior psychiatric illness was rare. More often than not the patient herself did not consider herself psychiatrically ill and sought a psychiatrist only upon the direction of an obstetrician. Although they stress the need of follow-up to avoid the psychological consequences of either approved or denied abortion, neither their own experience nor that of others would suggest that there are any particular emotional hazards involved. They found adverse reactions to be rare and in general, women were content with having had the abortion and felt themselves benefited by it. This accords with the experience of Kerslake in England who, on a mail follow-up, found 96 per cent of some 400 patients did not regret the procedure and had no psychological repercussions.[7]

Facts Replacing Beliefs

Improved statistical data is one of the most important consequences of the new Act in Britain, Colorado, and those states which have liberalized the law. Already facts accruing from these areas, especially Britain, lay to rest some of the dogmas that Pohlman assails in this issue. Polemic and iconoclastic, he uses a lancet rather than the curette he promises to dissect our cherished misbeliefs. Like doubting the Holy Grail, he even questions psychiatric judgment. He bustles with research suggestions only a few of which are touched upon in the following pages. At the rate laws are being changed many of his questions could soon be answered. Hopefully there will not be the same urgent need to do so as at present—changed practice will have rendered many of the dogmas he expounds extinct as the dodo.

REFERENCES

1. Aitken-Swan, J.: Some social characteristics on women seeking abortion. J. Biosoc. Sci. (in press).

2. Diggory, P., Peel, J., and Potts, M.: Preliminary assessment of the 1967 Abortion Act in practice. Lancet 1:287, 1970.

3. Finch, S. M.: Impact on children's mental health of unwanted status or crowded families. In Family planning and mental health: summary of discussion held at National Institute of Health, Washington, D.C.: Population Crisis Committee, 1966, pp. 7-8.

4. Friedan, Betty: Abortion: A woman's civil right. Keynote speech: First National Conference for Repeal of Abortion Laws, Chicago, Ill, February 14, 1969.

5. Reguena, M.: Studies of family planning in the Quinta Normal District of Santiago. Milbank Mem. Fund Quar., 43:69, 1965.

6. Karim, S. M. M., and Filshie, G. M.: Therapeutic abortion using prostglandin F_{2X}. Lancet, January 24, 1970.

7. Kerslake, D.: Preliminary report on psychological repercussions following termi-

nation of pregnancy. (Unpublished paper.)

8. Lamm, R.: Colorado: The law. Current Medical Digest, September 1969, p. 761.

9. —: Flaws in abortion reform found in an 8-state study. Quoted in McFadden, R. D. article in New York Times, April 13, 1970, p. 1.

10. MacGillivray, I.: Abortion in the North-East of Scotland. J. Biosoc. Sci. (in press).

11. Milhaven, J. G.: The abortion debate: an epistemological interpretation. Theological Studies, 31:106-124, 1970.

12. Pohlman, E.: The Psychology of Birth Planning. Cambridge, Mass., Schenkman Publishing, 1969.

13. Group for the Advancement of Psychiatry: GAP The Right to Abortion: A Psychiatric View. Formulated by the Committee of Psychiatry and Law, Vol. 7, No. 75, October 1969.

14. Rossi, A. E.: Abortion and social change. Dissent, July-August, 1969, pp. 338-346.

15. Vaillant, A. G.: The abortion problem: A woman's view. (unpublished paper).

R. Bruce Sloane, M.D.

Abortion Dogmas Needing Research Scrutiny

By EDWARD POHLMAN, PH.D.

T HE TOPIC OF ABORTION is undesirably swollen with dogmatic beliefs. Careful research may permit a dilation and curettage of those
dogmas that are unsubstantiated. The list below is illustrative, not complete.
Most of these dogmas involve so many variables that it is easy to draw wrong
conclusions, especially if one is equipped with preconceptions. Research and
interpretation of research should use proper controls for such factors as the
time in pregnancy when abortion is performed, setting in which performed
(hospital or clinic or physician's office or other locale), emergency supplies
available, training of person doing the operation, experience (in abortion) of
person performing the abortion, type of operation done (D & C, vacuum,
saline, etc.), culture and subculture in which performed, personal characteristics of patient (socioeconomic, psychological, health, etc.) and of person
performing operation, and previous history of physical and psychiatric problems. Few studies have been adequately controlled, and good studies are
often generalized indiscriminantly to other populations, including very different cultures where they are not necessarily applicable.

Our objective is to challenge belief on each dogma, not to work out details
of how research should proceed in checking the dogma. Also, we are not
claiming to present a systematic or critical review of existing literature on
these topics, but to provide enough leads to references, often through listing
other secondary sources, that the interested scholar can find the relevant
studies.

In addition to other papers published with this one, there are a number
of sources that list many studies of abortion,[1,4,8,22,23,28] but the would-be re-
searcher should consult the original studies. The reviewer typically cannot
condense all the crucial material and is perhaps inevitably biased by his own
feelings about abortion. As an example, one study[7] came out with the "right"
answers but wth poor methodology; it is cited repeatedly with no mention
that the control group contained far fewer out-of-wedlock births. One reviewer
even speaks of these controls as "matched very carefully" when no matching
was attempted. Reviewers are often in a hurry to produce another publication
and are insufficiently critical and thorough.

A major consideration in most evaluations of abortion is the need to compare abortion with results of not carrying it out, such as death, illness, emotional upset and sterility resulting from pregnancy which the abortion avoids;
population congestion; effects on the child born after abortion is denied, etc.

Dogma 1. Hospital abortion is dangerous to the mother's life. The dangers
of abortion must be specified in comparison to the dangers of carrying the
baby to a full term delivery.

Tietze[25] offers these death rates: approximately 3 per 100,000 hospital abortions in nations where physicians are experienced in abortion and abortion is

typically done early in pregnancy; approximately 20 per 100,000 in the U.S. from problems associated with pregnancy, birth, etc., excluding abortion. Thus it appears far safer to have an early expert abortion than to carry on with the pregnancy. The above low rates for abortion are based on over ten million abortions studied in Japan and Europe.[24,26] Scandinavian and U.S. deaths associated with abortion are higher; in these countries abortion is more difficult to get and those receiving it are more likely to face high medical risks and to have the operation performed after the twelfth week, when different abortive procedures are often used and risks are somewhat higher. Also, U.S. physicians performing abortions have typically had much less training and experience in the techniques than Japanese or East European counterparts.

Dogma 2. Hospital abortion is medically dangerous to the mother's physical health. The data available on this question is much less satisfactory because death is a more clear-cut criterion and more readily comparable from records.[24] There is no systematic evidence that hospital abortion produces any more problems for physical health than the continued pregnancy and birth which abortion avoids; the reverse may well be true.

Dogma 3. Abortion produces lowered reproductive capacity or sterility. These problems are often attributed to repeated abortions. An example of supposed problems is cervical inadequacy leading to miscarriages. A recent World Health Organization group concluded that evidence to prove this dogma in any of its variations has not been presented.[24] There is some association, they concluded, between prematurity and previous abortion, with the association being high with higher numbers of previous abortions.

Dogma 4. Illegal abortion is dangerous to the mother's life. Sometimes the party line of the "liberals" is that hospital abortion is safe, but illegal abortion outside of hospitals is extremely dangerous; hence full legalization of abortion would avoid many deaths from illegal abortion. Tietze[24] suggests that in some communities of the world deaths reach or exceed 1000 per 100,000 illegal abortions, but that in most countries as a whole risks are much lower. Where qualified physicians perform the illegal abortions and if there is ready access to satisfactory hospital care, Tietze sees even 50-100 deaths as possibly a high estimate. He sees the estimate of 5000 to 10,000 U.S. deaths annually from illegal abortion, based on evidence of some 30 years ago, as ridiculously high; he views the true total as not much above 400 per year. The major public health impact of illegal abortion in the U.S. is now no longer in terms of mortality but health and human dignity, argues Tietze.

Dogma 5. Oral contraception represents the safest way of birth control if the aim is to avoid almost all unwanted births. Using maternal deaths as the criterion of safety, Tietze[25] has estimated that there would be several times fewer deaths if one used contraceptive methods that had slightly more accidental pregnancies, combined with abortion to "mop up" the errors. Such methods would include pills with lower dosages than those currently used, as well as IUD's (intrauterine devices) and methods developed earlier.

Dogma 6. Abortion frequently produces psychiatric disturbance. This dogma has been supported by case studies. More systematic studies have been attempted but most have severe methodological flaws; we have listed only a few examples, with more stress on reviews of literature,[1,4,6,14,15,21,22,23,28] Reviews of the literature do not give consistent support to the dogma. Emotional upset experienced by some after abortion must be balanced against emotional upset[27] and psychiatric illness during and following the pregnancy which is carried to completion if there is no abortion. In abortion studies of psychiatric upset associated with either abortion or pregnancy, attention should be paid to the previous history of psychiatric disturbance before conception.

Dogma 7. Abortion frequently produces severe guilt. This dogma is related to the preceding, but deserves special attention. We hypothesize that the more tolerant the attitude of culture and subculture toward abortion (including its formal legislative stance), the less the guilt and the less the psychiatric disturbance to those women having abortion.

Dogma 8. Failure to get a desired abortion hurts mothers. This is a dogma of the liberals who favor liberalization or removal of anti-abortion legislation. We have argued above that results of abortion in terms of maternal death, ill health, sterility, psychiatric disturbance and milder emotional upset should be compared with paralled effects of the pregnancies which abortions prevent. Most of the discussions and studies which have stumbled toward conclusions on this point have compared abortions with pregnancies in general. However, it is possible that those who want abortions do so because they feel the urgency of more problems than other pregnant women. If so, using the latter as a control or comparison may underestimate the damage done by refusing abortion.

Two Swedish studies provide an example of the complex and sometimes confusing research. Most of a group of women refused abortion seemed to be upset,[10] but most of a group whose abortion requests had been formally approved but then not implemented with abortion were contented with the way things worked out.[2] In another study of those who had had abortions, 95 per cent said abortion was the answer to their problem.[14] It seems that whatever happens, there is some tendency to rationalize it as for the best, although this may conceal severe problems.

Domga 9. Mothers' failure to get a desired abortion hurts children. A liberal dogma parallel to Dogma 8, this one stresses that the child born when parents really wanted abortion (but failed to get it) is disadvantaged in comparison to appropriate controls. Siblings are also supposed to be disadvantaged. This dogma may be laid onto the foundation of economic hardship, space congestion, or maternal health. Often, however, it is phrased in terms of psychological reactions to maternal rejection. As such it becomes a specific subdivision of the broad general dogma that unwanted conceptions are "bad," a dogma that was a major war-cry of the planned parenthood movements. Careful reviews of available research find little evidence that unwanted conceptions are in a worse light than other (control) conceptions,

although this is primarily the result of inadequate and inconclusive, rather than negative, evidence.[16,17,19]

A Swedish study[7] claimed to find more problems among children whose mothers had been refused abortion than among controls. But the former contained 27 per cent born out of wedlock, as against 7.5 per cent for controls. This finding is presented as a dependent variable but substantially affects the independent variable. A reanalysis of data with controls for this factor would be useful. "Battered" and abused children, a focus of much recent medical interest, might be studied especially to see whether more of them were born after abortion was wanted (but not obtained) than among relevant controls.

Dogma 10. When women are refused abortion they adjust and learn to want the babies. This is part of the broader dogma that unwanted conceptions become wanted pregnancies and babies. More unwanted conceptions become wanted than vice versa, but by no means all make this shift, and even for those who do the principal logical explanation there seems to be rationalization and self-deception.[18]

Dogma 11. If necessary, children born after abortion is refused can always be given up for adoption. There are close to half a million children in institutions and temporary foster homes, and half of these are judged to be there because of parental neglect, abuse, or inability to care for offspring.[3,9] There is little adoption demand for any except very young attractive white babies; even for them the demand is no longer as great as it was. One or two temporary foster home placements, or a few months in an institution, often ruin a child's appeal for adoption.

Dogma 12. A live birth is a victory. If the woman can be "managed" through the pregnancy by drugs, psychotherapy, or other procedures so that she avoids a threatened spontaneous abortion, or gives up her request for induced abortion, the physician often feels that a victory has been achieved. Often he has few medical contacts with the woman or her children after delivery, knows little about the family's overall daily problems and way of living, and is not a specialist in population. Are there already several children who will be crowded and deprived by an additional baby? Does the acceptance of pregnancy last only until the woman gets home from the hospital, so that when the hand-holding encouragement or drugs or psychotherapy ends the baby is not wanted? Apparently, poverty-level families are chained to continue poverty partly by large families; small ones permit breaking these chains. But in considering a live birth a victory, there is a concentration on the present in blindness to the future, on the mother in blindness to the child, on the individual in contrast to society. Long-range research is needed, especially prospective research.

Dogma 13. Decisions on abortion requests should be made without respect to population problems. There is some dispute whether the U.S. already has an overpopulation problem, but few doubt that after a few decades there will be a severe one even in this country. The baby born when abortion requests are denied does not merely add to population now; on the average, he will be alive for threescore years and ten and add to crowding at a time when, according to present forecasts, congestion will be alarming. Also, he will probably have children of his own and multiply his role as a "crowder" forever. Traditionally, medical ethics have stressed saving and conserving every human life possible, and the well-being of the individual rather than the group. But population problems may warrant some reexamination. If mothers do not want to continue pregnancy anyway, population factors might justifiably be taken into consideration in the physician's decision.

In many developing countries, such as India, there are almost none who doubt that we already have today an acute overpopulation problem. Yet the medical personnel in some of those countries, often with a Western-oriented tradition and rationale, refuse to allow population problems as a consideration in deciding whether to liberalize abortion laws and procedures.

Dogma 14. Psychiatrists can predict who will be disturbed by abortion. The custom of psychiatric referral rests in part on the assumption that psychiatric predictions have some degree of validity. To check this, a "double-blind study" might be done which would give psychiatric interviews to all applicants, and then lock up the decisions and opinions and keep them hidden from applicants and physicians handling the case. All applicants would be given abortion, regardless of (unknown) psychiatric opinion. Follow-up studies would then open the locked files and see how effectively the psychiatrists were able to predict which cases were going to have problems.

Dogma 15. Psychiatrists can predict more effectively than psychiatric social workers, clinical psychologists, secretaries or mothers. Following the research plan outlined under Dogma 14, patients could be seen by a number of different kinds of personnel, each of whom kept his opinions completely hidden from others. Follow-up studies would check the relative validity of predictions by various groups, to see whether the use of more costly and scarce personnel is justified.

Dogma 16. Interviews can predict more effectively than psychological tests. Following the research plan outlined under Dogma 14, a battery of psychological tests could be administered and predictive validity compared with that of interviews. Perhaps a "cutoff score" approach could be used, so that all those on one side of the cutoff would receive abortion without interviews, while dubious cases would be interviewed.

Dogma 17. Consultation by psychiatrists and psychologists, is needed. The whole necessity of interviewing and testing for psychiatric angles should be questioned, on several grounds. If research recommended under Dogmas 14, 15, and 16 shows poor predictive value, this throws psychiatric screening into doubt. Even if one can predict somewhat validly which woman will have disturbance after abortion, this does not mean she will have any less disturbance if pregnancy is allowed to continue; and it does not preclude the possibility that refusing abortion may do more eventual harm to humanity in terms of effects on an unwanted child, on siblings and fathers and family relationships, and on population. Psychiatric screening takes up valuable time and scarce manpower; if the volume of abortions grows greatly, as seems probable, this will be especially true. Psychiatric screening is not routinely demanded of any other surgical procedures, even though some of these, such as hysterectomy, lead to a certain proportion of subsequent disturbances. Certain European countries and Japan give abortion on a massive scale with no routine psychiatric screening, without apparent national ill effects. If psychiatric approval of the abortion applicant is needed to reassure a nervous public and medical colleagues, especially during a time of transition, this might be given as a perfunctory rubber stamp. Routine screening costs patients money and this discriminates against the poor. If a woman has an inherent legal right to an abortion if she wants one, as some claim and certain court decisions seem to support, then psychiatric screening procedures may be an unjustified invasion of privacy. In practice the present screening procedures often involve protracted delays, shuttling of patients back and forth, condescension, and insults to dignity. Although these are characteristic of a fair proportion of medical practice in general, private but also especially public, they are especially true of abortion.

Psychiatric consultation arose historically as a welcome ruse and maneuver when psychiatric opinion was often the only way to sneak in a woman legally. But if this necessity changes, one may question the need for the routine procedure, especially if the judgments are to be made toward shortsighted and unbalanced criteria.

Dogma 18. Abortion is very expensive to society. If the claim were that abortion is much more expensive than contraception, this might seem obvious concerning many methods as used in many countries. But the dogma overlooks the comparative costs of pregnancy and delivery, and babies who grow up. Whether the easier availability of abortion makes people less vigilant about contraception and thus produces more pregnancies is itself a question for research (see a subsequent dogma), although there are strong reasons for doubting that it would have any such effect in the U.S. Research should compare costs of expert abortion early in pregnancy with those of pregnancy and delivery; the latter are probably much greater. Also, the child born after abortion is refused costs the tax-paying public in terms of education, public health, etc., and often welfare and institutionalization. Estimates of per-child costs to tax-payers in North Carolina[11] run into thousands of dollars. The "cost" dogma implies a cold economic calculation; if matters are put on this footing, it seems likely that abortion is an enormous bargain for society.

Dogma 19. Medical facilities and manpower are not adequate to take care of a large volume of abortions. Examination of this dogma exactly parallels the ideas listed at the start of the discussion of Dogma 18—the demands of pregnancies, which abortions can avoid, are probably much greater on scarce hospital space, medical manpower, and the like. For example, if obstetricians would spend more time on abortion, they would have to spend less time delivering babies. Potts[20] claimed that two abortions per week by each of the 660 obstetrician-gynecologists practicing in England and Wales would easily handle the case load which is sometimes portrayed as deluging the entire profession. Thus even aside from the reduction in deliveries which abortions could bring about, volume is not so enormous, if it were distributed equally among relevant practitioners who find abortion ethically acceptable.

Dogma 20. Abortion must be paid for privately. Among poor people, pregnancy and delivery costs are sometimes paid by public funds; why not abortions? Since those performing abortions want to be compensated, and poor people on welfare are often unable to make the heavy payments required, is discrimination implied? Only recently a similar point has been made concerning contraception, and the policy of government support for contraceptive services and supplies (as acceptable to the individual's beliefs and as requested by them when offered) has been accepted. Can a parallel policy be developed concerning abortion? If not, it is probable that the poor will continue to have a sharply exaggerated share of illegal abortions, incompetently done abortions, medical complications and deaths from abortions, and defective children born after unsuccessful attempts at abortion.

Dogma 21. Only physicians should perform abortions. Paramedical personnel are being used in some countries.[1] Comparative data on the safety and effectiveness of medical and paramedical personnel performing abortions is needed, with appropriate controls. In the U.S., research on possibilities of well-trained midwives and nurses doing abortion is needed. It is ironic that in some parts of the U.S., midwives are allowed to deliver babies because of the scarcity of physicians, but although births are more dangerous than early abortions, they are not allowed to perform abortions which might prevent unwanted and more dangerous births, despite a parallel scarcity of physicians to perform abortions.[1]

Dogma 22. Abortion must be a complicated medical procedure. The development of an acceptably safe and effective oral abortifacient or other simple procedure would alter many of the previously correct generalizations about abortion. Even the vacuum method has had this effect.

Dogma 23. Liberalization or repeal of abortion legislation will automatically increase number of abortions substantially. In several states with recent liberalization in abortion legislation, the expected massive increase in abortions and the expected greater ease with which women could find abortions have not appeared.[1] Abortion boards often provide a group behind which refusals can be hidden, cost money, and may mean a reduction in the number of abortions a hospital performs. Many of the restraints on more general availability of abortion appear to spring from within the structures of the medical profession rather than from laws of the society.

Dogma 24. Ready availability of legal abortion will decrease illegal abortion. Two thoughtful discussions of this question[5,13] provide no consistent overall pattern; it seems that the answer has varied from country to country, and the "stage" in social change of a country. In East Germany[12] liberalizing legislation appeared to result in an increase of both legal and illegal abortions. The greater availability of legal abortion probably stimulates a general desire to avoid unwanted children, and makes family planning more visible and fashionable. The preference for illegal rather than legal abortions can be explained by the greater privacy, lesser red tape, and greater speed with which illegal abortion can sometimes be obtained.

Brackett[5] stresses that East Germany may well be an exception, with particular social chaos in the postwar period and the high rates of pre-marital pregnancy that social disorder so often produces, and other unique factors. Data from other countries suggest that legalization may reduce illegal abortion.

Perhaps a more important question is whether increased availability of legal abortion increases the overall quality of all abortions that are performed (legal and illegal combined). It appears that in some European countries where a tolerant view is taken of physicians' performing of technically illegal abortions, the illegal abortions are done primarily by experts and are quite safe. The-oretically, the competition should drive out the clumsy bunglers responsible for poor quality in abortion; if women are attracted to the slightly greater privacy and speed of illegal abortions, this will be primarily if they perceive the safety and other considerations to be about equal. Restrictive abortion policies probably encourage poor quality in illegal abortion while permissive policies have the reverse effect.

Dogma 25. Illegal abortion is always incompetent, dangerous and undesir-able. The preceding section is relevant to this dogma. In the U.S., many of the illegal abortions are performed by fully trained, accredited and re-spected physicians, whose medical practices may be completely legal except when they help women avoid unwanted births by performing abortions.

Dogma 26. Society must decide whether abortion is morally "right" or "wrong." Repeal of prohibition against drinking alcohol was not accom-plished in the U.S. by a societal decision that drinking was "right" but merely by the concept that each individual should be allowed to decide for himself. Concerning theft and murder, society takes the view that the individual does not have the right to make up his mind about whether it is right. Many view abortion as in the same category. The strategy need not be to convince them that abortion is morally "right," but only that it is like drinking alcohol (and not like stealing): it is a matter for individual choice in a pluralistic society.

Those who believe abortion to be "right" are not interested in forcing women or physicians who believe it is "wrong" to participate in it against their will. But neither do they wish to be denied abortion—with a resulting forced childbearing for women against their will—by those who view it as "wrong."

Dogma 27. Availability of abortion increases out-of wedlock intercourse, both among married people having affairs and unmarried youth. This dogma is parallel to the similar one about contraception; in the early days of con-traception it was argued that it would decrease marital fidelity; this was recently voiced again concerning the pill and IUD; and it is widely argued that contraception available to the unmarried or promoted among them will increase premarital intercourse. Research on these dogmas is needed.

Dogma 28. Contraception, if available, will reduce abortion. This may depend heavily on the country and subculture in question and the stage in "family planning development." There is some reason, as well as some empirical evidence, to suggest the opposite effect, at least on a short-run basis.[13] If contraception whets appetite for capacity to control family size, raising hopes for planned families, but meanwhile if contraception is not completely successful, the disappointed may turn to abortion. Some have hypothesized that societies tend to pass through phases, with contraception initially producing increases in abortion, eventually followed by decreases as contraception becomes more expertly practiced and effective and replaces abortion to a larger extent.

Dogma 29. Abortion will reduce/increase contraception. The increased availability of abortion will make people less vigilant in contraception; or, alternatively, will lead them to want better birth planning methods. We know of no controlled research on this question.

Dogma 30. Abortion is the most common method of birth control in the world. Perhaps it would not be fruitful to try to test this oft-heard dogma with research, since the relevant evidence is so well hidden in many cases. But at least this should be recognized as opinion rather than as research conclusion.

Dogma 31. Abortion is used primarily by the married/the single. One hears both versions. To combat the bad image of abortion as a back-alley remedy for illicit sex, liberals have sometimes claimed in recent years that the bulk of abortions serve mothers overburdened by large families. Fragmentary data concerning states with newly liberalized abortion policies call this liberal dogma in question, however. Perhaps the answer is heavily specific to country, subculture, time and even hospital or physician.

Dogma 32. Men are not affected by abortion. Attitudes, role, influence, and effects on males, whether husbands, lovers, ex-boyfriends, fathers in incest cases, etc., need exploration with research.

Dogma 33. Blacks use abortion more than whites. Applied primarily to the U.S., this vague dogma may reflect a prejudice and as such not be precisely specified. It appears that on a per capita basis middle class women and whites have in the past been given more of the benefits of hospital abortion, but deaths from illegal abortion are higher among blacks. Neither kind of material indicates that blacks make more use of abortion per se.

Dogma 34. Economic reasons are the primary ones for desiring abortion. This dogma makes good public relations for abortion. Unfortunately research to support this dogma is often worthless because financial limitations are often a "noble" reason to give, whatever the real reasons, for wanting abortion or even for not wanting to conceive additional children.[16] Also, some recent surveys noted that the majority of women did not mention this as their reason, despite its convenience as a possible rationalization.[1]

Summary

Dogmas hold that abortion is expensive to society, medically dangerous, psychologically dangerous, and that it produces sterility and guilt; that failure to get desired abortion hurts mothers, families, and children, or is followed by acceptance of the baby, or adoption; that abortion does not relate to overpopulation or men; that psychiatric screening is superior to standarized tests and is routinely necessary; that abortion must be done by a physician. These and many other dogmas about abortion—some of them "liberal dogmas"—need research scrutiny. Effects of abortion must be compared with effects of pregnancy and birth on mothers, families, social mental health, and population.

REFERENCES

1. Abortion, Obtained and Denied: Research Approaches to Outcomes. Studies in Fam. Plan. 53:1–8, 1970.

2. Aren, P., and Amark, C.: The prognosis in cases in which legal abortion has been granted but not carried out. Acta Psychiatrica et Neurologica Scandinavica 36: 203-278, 1961.

3. Beck, M. B.: Abortion: the mental health consequences of unwantedness. Sem. Psych. 2:263–274, 1970.

4. —, Newman, S. H., and Tietze, S.: Abortion: a national public and mental health problem—past, present and proposed research. Amer. J. Pub. Health (in press).

5. Brackett, J. W.: The demographic consequences of legal abortion. Studies in Fam. Plan. 53:6, 1970.

6. Ekblad, M.: Induced abortion on psychiatric grounds: a follow-up study of 479 women. Acta Psychiatrica et Neurologica Scandinavica, supplement 99: 1-238, 1955.

7. Forssman, H., and Thuwe, I.: One hundred and twenty children born after application for therapeutic abortion refused. Acta Psychiat. Scand. 42:71-88, 1966.

8. afGeijerstam, G. K.: An Annotated Bibliography of Induced Abortion. Ann Arbor, Mich., Univ. of Mich. Center for Population Planning, 1968.

9. Haitch, R.: Orphans of the Living: The Foster Care Crisis. Washington, U.S. Children's Bureau Public Affairs Pamphlet No. 418, published in cooperation with the Child Welfare League of America, 1968.

10. Hook, K.: Refused abortion: a follow-up study of 249 women whose applications were refused by the National Board of Health in Sweden. Acta Psychiat. Scand. 39: 1-156, 1963.

11. Leasure, J. W.: Some economic benefits of birth prevention. Milbank Mem. Fund Quart. 45:417–425, 1967.

12. Mehlan, K. H. (Ed.): Internationale Abortsituation, Abortbekampfung, Antikonzeption. Liepzig, Georg Thieme, 1961, pp. 55-60.

13. Moore, E. C.: Induced abortion and contraception. Studies in Fam. Plan. 53: 7–8, 1970.

14. Niswander, K. R., and Patterson, R. J.: Psychologic reaction to therapeutic abortion. Obstet. Gynec. 29:702–706, 1967.

15. Peck, A., and Marcus, H.: Psychiatric sequelae of therapeutic interruption of pregnancy. J. Nerv. Ment. Dis. 143:417-425, 1966.

16. Pohlman, E.: The Psychology of Birth Planning. Cambridge, Mass., Schenkman, 1969.

17. —: Children born after abortion requests are refused. Studies in Fam. Plan. 53:4–5, 1970.

18. —: Changes from rejection to acceptance of pregnancy. Soc. Sci. Med. 2:337-340, 1968.

19. —: Unwanted conceptions: Research on undesirable consequences. Eugen. Quart. 14:143-154, 1967.

20. Potts, M.: Informal presentation at Planned Parenthood-World Population, New York, October, 1969. Cited by Moore.[13]

21. Simon, N. M.: Psychological and emotional indications for therapeutic abortion. Sem. Psych. 2:283–301, 1970.

22. —, and Senturia, A.: Psychiatric sequelae of abortion: review of the literature, 1935-1964. Arch. Gen. Psychiat. 15: 378-389, 1966.

23. Sloane, R. B.: The unwanted pregnancy. New Eng. J. Med. 280:1213, 1969.

24. Tietze, C.: Somatic consequences of abortion. Studies in Fam. Plan. 53:2-3, 1970.

25. —: Mortality with contraception and induced abortion. Studies in Fam. Plan.

45:6-8, 1969.

26. —, and Lehfeldt, H.: Legal abortion in Eastern Europe. JAMA 175:1149–1154, 1969.

27. Tobin, S. M.: Emotional depression during pregnancy. Obstet. Gynec. 10:677-681, 1957.

28. Wolff, S. R.: Therapeutic abortion: a liaison psychiatrist's perspective. Studies in Fam. Plan. 53:4, 1970.

To Whom Does the Child Belong?

By Alan A. Stone, M.D., Milton Greenblatt, M.D., Jack Ewalt, M.D.,
and William Curran, L.L.M., Sc.M.

D R. GREENBLATT: When asked for a way to organize a discussion on
the GAP report, I suggested the topic "To Whom Does the Child Belong?" as basically a moral issue. But if we could get the answer to that
question, it might throw light on other bothersome issues. We would also
like a few words from Alan on how this report evolved.

Dr. Stone: I found that in the preparation of the report as one really looks
into the criteria for abortion and as one looks at the liberalization of the
laws in most states and the more generous interpretation of the statutes, one
finds that there are more abortions being performed and almost always on
psychiatric grounds. So that as legal abortion is increasing, the major justification for the increase is on psychiatric grounds. Then, as one goes through
the literature trying to find if there has ever been any sort of controlled study
or even any careful clinical studies of the criteria for abortion on psychiatric
grounds, one finds there never was a controlled study and that in questionnaire studies, psychiatrists were operating by the seat of their pants: that
some were being very generous and others very conservative. This did not
seem to reflect any stable body of clinical knowledge, but rather the psychiatrists' own values. The lawyers who studied this looked at the different
hospitals and the different psychiatrists and were struck by the fantastic
differences in hospital practices, and doctor practices, which clearly began
to raise issues from the legal point of view of due process.

That kind of information played an important part in the recent District
of Columbia decision where Judge Gesell, who is, by the way, son of the
pediatrician Dr. Arnold Gesell, declared that the law was unconstitutionally
vague and impinged on certain rights of the woman and the doctor. Therefore, the first thing we should face is that the psychiatric criteria for abortion
are nowhere near as hard as we would like and are being misinterpreted
by psychiatrists or misunderstood or whatever. As Louisell pointed out, this
was not all the psychiatrists' fault: the law is difficult to interpret.

Another important concern is that abortion does psychic harm to women.
There have been psychoanalytic notions that there was always guilt, having
murdered someone, and so on. But when one looked into the good, careful
follow-up studies by people like Simon of St. Louis and his group, one
found that when a woman is motivated for abortion, the psychiatric sequelae
seemed really minimal and one had to face the possibility that an event

---

*Shortly after the release of the most recent publication from the Group for the Advancement of Psychiatry (GAP)—The Right to Abortion: A Psychiatric View—Alan A.
Stone, Milton Greenblatt, Jack Ewalt, and William Curran met to discuss several aspects
of the report. This article is a transcript of their discussion.*

21

that might be etched on somebody's soul could, from the symptomatic point of view, not cause grave psychiatric harm.

Based on these kinds of considerations, I became convinced that at least on the psychiatric evidence one's burden was to tell the public that the psychiatrist should not take on this role of deciding who should be aborted because he can not do it with the kind of authority that society thinks he can. And, second, the idea that abortion causes serious depression and perhaps is a focus for involutional melancholia does not seem to be demonstrated in terms of what we now know.

Would you like me to go further in terms of your question "To whom does the child belong?" Obviously, the people to consider are the mother, the father, the child himself and the state in some way.

I think Father Drinan, Dean of the Boston College Law School, has made the argument as to the issue of the child in a most coherent fashion. As a legal scholar, he does not present the argument in such simple terms as "to whom does the child belong." He starts looking at "rights" and it's quite clear that the unborn child does have a number of rights, such as the right to inherit if his father dies before he is born. He also has the right to sue, the right not to be harmed by drugs. He has the right to bring a tort action. For example, if his mother takes thalidomide, the child or the mother, when the baby is eventually born, can sue. If the mother is in an accident and there is some damage to the unborn child, again he can sue. There are thus certain legal rights, and on this basis one can extend the argument and say he also has a right to a life of his own. That is the kind of argument Father Drinan has made and it is a major legal and ethical issue.

The greatest practical problem, in contrast, is the father. It is true that in the past most criminal abortions were being done on married women with about three children. But in the last few years, the picture has changed so that at least half of the criminal abortions are being done on young girls, unmarried, where the father is either a boyfriend or some casual acquaintance or in other ways does not have an important emotional relationship with the woman. What has already happened in the legal sphere is that a father brought a tort action against the doctor who performed an abortion on his wife on the basis that he had been deprived of his child. Now, he did not win the case but at least the judge considered that this might at some point be a possibility.

Dr. Ewalt: May I ask a legal question? Suppose a father is killed in an accident and his wife is three weeks to a month pregnant. His will leaves half the money to his wife and half to be divided among his children. Does that unborn child inherit his due share? Does he have rights as early as one month?

Dr. Stone: Yes. He has the right to inherit.

Dr. Ewalt: Then you are in a difficult spot to justify any abortion. If he has the right to inherit, then under the law he is a human being.

Dr. Greenblatt: But when do the rights occur? Do they occur right after conception?

Dr. Stone: If a baby is born nine, perhaps even ten, months after the father's death, he would still be entitled to inheritance.

Dr. Greenblatt: So when they do an abortion, they are killing a potential heir?

Prof. Curran: That is right. And they are killing a potential tort-suit bringer.

Dr. Greenblatt: So then the infant's right to inherit starts right after conception. Suppose a mother was pregnant for six or seven months and decided to abort and accomplished this by battering the child somehow. Let us say the child was born with several broken ribs, or something of that sort, what would be the posture of the law in this case?

Dr. Stone: The striking thing about abortion is that it is one form of murder, if you want to call it murder, in which the principal is almost never prosecuted. The one who gets prosecuted is the abortionist, who does it at the request of the mother. There are statutes, but as far as I have been able to find out, charges against the mother are almost never pressed. In the large Los Angeles hospitals, they have up to fifty women a day coming in after a self-induced or criminal abortion and none of them are prosecuted.

Dr. Ewalt: The thing that bothers me is the question "to whom does the child belong." No one belongs to anybody but himself. He may be a member of a family and the family may be responsible for him, but he still belongs to himself.

Dr. Greenblatt: I do not agree with that. You belong to yourself only to a limited degree. There are many things you can not do to yourself that you may want to. You are constricted in your own control of your own actions.

Dr. Ewalt: Only as they relate to the rights of other people. I have a right to take my own life.

Prof. Curran: The point you have all been making is that one has to think in terms of rights and responsibilities, rather than in terms of ownership. It seems to me from my investigation into this, that the law has been functioning in the opposite direction. Doctors are now giving young girls a legal abortion if the girl can demonstrate that she has an independent household, that is, if she is independently domiciled, even if she is only 18 years old. In some states they will not even require her to notify her parents if she is about to have an abortion. And of course there are all sorts of judgments which favor her not having to expose her private sexual life at this point to her parents, again even if she is only 18. The test in some ways would be if she is independent in terms of where she is living, going to school or working. It is then that the parents do not have to be involved.

Dr. Stone: I do not think we have yet dealt with the problem of the father sufficiently. Let me give you an example. Suppose I am 55-years-old and I am a practicing Catholic and marry a younger woman who is Catholic but not devout. I have not had any children. I then get my wife pregnant. We have a fight and she is angry. She did not want to have a baby anyway and now she wants to have an abortion. What right do I have? Here perhaps is my only possible heir. Not only that, but I am a Catholic and feel very strongly about abortion. This seems to me is the toughest kind of situation.

Prof. Curran: We are at the brink of a strong possibility that we will soon have a Supreme Court decision which will totally affect the whole situation if it at all takes a view similar to that of the lower court. Now, this is on the right of privacy, on the right of the woman.

I think from the psychiatric viewpoint, there should be explorations of the woman's problem of guilt afterward or of the issues of when a physician should recommend abortion, or if we do accept the fact that we may well have changes in the law, how the physician should behave under changed conditions. I am firmly in support of this kind of review because I have always been against the American Law Institute (ALI) proposal.[1]* If we get major changes in the law, it seems to me necessary to place the physician in his proper role as a physician concerned only with the interests of his patient. (You talk the law, Alan, and I shall talk medicine— we shall reverse our roles.) It seems to me there would be a very different legal question when the woman is married. There is a long medical history involving both husband and wife in marital decisions.

In discussing the law at present without a Supreme Court decision, we have the great problem of examining the different laws in the different states.

Dr. Stone: As far as I know in no state does the father have a right.

Prof. Curran: Well, I think these are the kinds of issues that are new and can and should be discussed. I do not know of any siituation where a lawyer would recommend that a married woman get an abortion without involving the husband and without getting his permission. We do not advise on the basis of the law the Supreme Court may make in the future. We advise on what we judge the law to be now and we advise getting the husband's consent in order to prevent a lawsuit and all the discomfort, publicity, and embarrassment it might entail.

Dr. Greenblatt: Suppose the woman is recently separated from her husband and gets pregnant by someone else? She is not divorced, she is still legally married.

Prof. Curran: Here in Massachusetts, we certainly always advise the physician to act under legal counsel. We always ask him to put a letter into his file indicating this. We try to get a clear indication of what kind of separation it is and what the problem is. In general, we would recommend that if it is the child of some other man and not the husband, the woman should go ahead without the husband's consent. We will always at-

---

*ALI proposal: A licensed physician is justified in terminating a pregnancy if:

(a) he believes there is substantial risk that continuance of the pregnancy would gravely impair the physical or mental health of the mother or that the child would be born with grave physical or mental defect, or the pregnancy resulted from rape or force or its equivalent as defined in Section 207.4(1) or from incest as defined in Section 207.3; and

(b) two physicians, one of whom may be the person performing the abortion, have certified in writing their belief in the justifying circumstances, and have filed such certificate prior to the abortion in the licensed hospital where it was to be performed, or in such other place as may be designated by law.

tempt to protect her, but again, legally. We will advise the physician on how he can act. This is a separate question from telling him what the law is. If I were advising a physician, I would not be as much inclined to tell him what the law is, as to tell him what I would advise him to do in order to protect himself.

Dr. Greenblatt: Yes, but you are still talking about the current law, where the excuse for abortion is some illness in the mother.

Prof. Curran: A great majority of states suppose danger to the woman. Massachusetts as you know is one of the more liberal states in having psychiatric grounds.

Dr. Greenblatt: You say you subscribe to this point of view. Does this mean that you reject the position of the Catholic church?

Prof. Curran: As far as law is concerned, yes. The position of religion is not necessarily of significance as to what the law should be.

Dr. Greenblatt: Now with this point of view, we are taking what I think is a simplistic view in terms of procedure, that is, we leave it to the mother. That is a lot less vague in many ways than using the ALI criteria. We leave to the mother a very profound decision, whether she has an IQ of 60 or 160.

Prof. Curran: We are being simplistic. We are leaving it to the mother and hoping that the decision on an abortion will be made in a medical setting with good medical advice.

Dr. Greenblatt: I shall come to that in a moment. But we are leaving it to the mother. You pointed out a broad spectrum of interpretation of what we have got now. I agree. From what little I have heard, one hospital will never do abortions and another hospital three blocks away will always do them.

Dr. Stone: I am not sure that will change.

Prof. Curran: I suspect too that it will not change because the religious issues and other things will remain. Removing a law does not necessarily change the religious factor.

Dr. Stone: Judge Gesell in the District of Columbia decision specifically indicated that he expected that the municipal hospitals and so forth in the District of Columbia would do something about their relative lack of therapeutic abortions.

Dr. Greenblatt: Here we have a wide disparity in ways of interpreting what we now have. Then we leave it to the woman, which as I say makes it much easier for many people. You meet young people with varying IQs, varying motivations, different ages, and different family settings. Some of them are neurotic or semipsychotic. Probably many of them have real character disorders. Their motivations for abortions will be the thinnest and the least mature. It boggles the imagination what they will do. Maybe becoming pregnant might be just a pure act of hostility of some kind on a flimsy basis and they want to go through abortion after abortion.

Where we have yielded is a simpler solution which looks easier because it respects more the rights of the woman. It does away with a lot of the illegality, etc. We have not really squared it with the issues of today. What are the rights and responsibilities of *all parties* involved? If the decision were that the rights and responsibilities were somehow distributed then you would have to bring all the individuals into consideration.

Dr. Stone: Prof. Curran has, I think, an important point and I would like to persevere with it. He is saying that he was against ALI, as I was and that we have the prospect of considerable change. It seems as though, if there is a change, that it will still involve and be administered by the medical establishment. This is one problem. Another is what I think we are going to see in the future. If the Supreme Court strikes down these abortion statutes as unconstitutionally vague, then I think one of the things the legislatures will immediately do is try to draft statutes that are not vague.

Prof. Curran: I think it would be wrong for the court to strike them down on that basis because they would open the door for tighter statutes.

Dr. Stone: If they do strike them down on that basis, then all of us are going to be involved in legislative hearings and so forth in terms of how to draft clearer statutes from a medical point of view. But if we do turn in the direction of abortion being the right of the woman, then I think we should look at what has happened in some of the eastern European countries where although abortion on request was not the right of the woman, it was fairly easy to get an abortion. What happened there is that the rate of abortions went up to such a degree that if one transposed their experience to the American scene, we would be apt to have up to 3½ million therapeutic abortions a year, compared with approximately 4½ million children being born each year. If we behaved like the Japanese, we would have about 2½ million abortions a year.

Things got so bad in some of the eastern European countries that the Ob-Gyn residents went on strike. They were in there all day long performing abortions. They were offended as human beings by it. Political reaction developed when the population actually started to shrink in size. I am told now that in Greece the population is beginning to shrink on the basis of illegal abortions, not legal abortions.

There is no doubt in my mind that if we went to abortion on request, there would be a profound effect. Furthermore, it is very hard to give women rights legally when you still have a social structure in which men call the shots. So you might say that now it is the woman who has the right. But take a young couple. The husband may very well say, "Well, I'd like you to have an abortion because you've got this marvelous job and you're working my way through graduate school." There is some speculation that these factors operated in Japan and eastern Europe. I am not at all sure that the kind of legal solution of leaving abortions up to the woman will in reality leave it up to the woman.

Dr. Greenblatt: When you leave it up to the woman, you are leaving the right of self-determination up to her. Then you have to make a law that defines the exercise of this right. For example, the woman says, "I want to have an abortion." Is she competent to make this judgment about herself? She might be psychotic and so we would still have the vagaries of judgment as to competence and so forth.

Dr. Stone: If she is psychotic, it seems to me that she can probably get an abortion on the old grounds.

Dr. Ewalt: In terms of really being able to get a legal abortion, there is no current real reason to change the law now. If a woman comes forward and says that she wants an abortion, one must make sure that she is doing this of her own free will and not under coercion, such as when the husband says that she is working his way through graduate school or her mother says "you're disgracing our family and you'll never be able to get a good husband if you have had an illegitimate child." This has been a crucial issue in a number of cases. A girl might say she wants an abortion and you find out that it is not she who wants it but her mother or her grandmother or some other party.

Dr. Stone: I would agree with that wholeheartedly. That is the major problem in giving the right to the woman. How does she exercise that right without duress, undue duress from various sources?

Dr. Greenblatt: This right, is it really what she wants? She says she wants the abortion, but then after three interviews you and she find she really does not want it. It is a matter of clarification of motivations.

Prof. Curran: On this issue, perhaps we should examine the GAP recommendations.[2] It seems to me that the first sentence in "Summary and Recommendations" is entirely correct. The sentence is this: "It is on the basis of the foregoing discussion that we recommend an abortion, when performed by a licensed physician [note that] be entirely removed from the domain of criminal law." That is a perfectly acceptable statement. It is the second sentence that gets us in trouble: "We believe that a woman should have the right to abort or not, just as she has the right to marry or not."[2]

Now we are into this realm of "rights." Are we saying that the woman not only has a right, but she has a right to force the physician to perform the abortion even if after the three or so interviews or whatever he does, he makes a negative decision? Giving her the right, what kind of right is it? It is *not* the same as a right to marry. It is not the same as a right to vote. You see the loose use of words here. It seems to me that in the Supreme Court's use of the term "privacy," when it was examining the right to marry, it was saying that there shall not be laws against interracial marriage, and to that extent, people have a "right" to marry. That is, the state should not interfere with the decision of two people of different races to enter into marriage. In the earlier case—birth control—it was not really saying people have the "right" to use contraceptives; what it *was* saying is that it really is not any business of the criminal law, that the married couple is free to make the decision between themselves to use or not to use a contraceptive. I do not think they were saying that if a husband forces his wife to use contraceptives and forces her almost in a rape situation that the law cannot have anything to do with that. That is not what the law was saying. It was just saying that as a matter of criminal law, we should not interfere with the voluntary actions of a married couple to decide to use contraceptives.

Dr. Ewalt: If you use that like a right to marry, then you are also saying that a woman has a right to demand plastic surgery or an appendectomy. She has neither of these rights. She has to scout around until she finds somebody who will agree with her and do it.

Prof. Curran: The second sentence still gives me pause.

Dr. Stone: That second sentence is clarified later on. It is made very clear subsequently that the doctor must be willing to do it and that the comparison is as you say to elective surgery. It is not that she can force a doctor to do it or she has a right to force a doctor to do it. I think Bill's clarification of rights is helpful but there is a remaining problem, and that pertains to municipal hospitals.

If you do a study and it turns out that there are twenty times more legal abortions done on private patients than on clinic patients, then that begins to be the kind of evidence that the law is being applied inequitably and that is what Judge Gesell was talking about. That is what the American Civil Liberties Union has emphasized and I think that is quite reasonable.

Prof. Curran: That is one of the reasons I was against the ALI proposal. It created situations where you had to make a medical situation almost a legal judgment. If you leave in the law processes and criteria by which decisions are made, you have to require that they be made in an equitable manner. In that sense, you almost have to reimpose a legal system to make sure that decisions are made equitably as to whom you will abort and whom you will not abort. But if you totally remove, as it says here, the criminal law, what is the continuing involvement of the law in question of poor and rich, which can be done in elective surgery right and left? It is hardly limited to the subject of abortion. In fact, the abortion might even be a higher scale than most of the other things. There are some social thinkers who would abort more of the poor than the rich, more of the black than the white, in order to reduce the population of the "undesirables."

Dr. Greenblatt: You say it is clarified later, but all that I find clarified is that medical judgment will be affected by factors such as length of gestation, viability of fetus, and maybe even motivation, etc. All that the clarification seems to me to mean is that the woman is going to live through it and be properly healthful and so on. But the point that you raise is not clarified by that. A woman comes and says, "Look, I'm at the proper gestational period, I have proper motivation, you've got to accept me for abortion." How do you avoid that?

Dr. Stone: Well I think you will see that it specifically says, although it is in a footnote, that a physician should have the right to refuse to perform an abortion on the basis of his own moral and religious conviction.

Dr. Greenblatt: How are you going to work that out? This is a *should*. I do not see any guidelines.

Dr. Stone: Also, in the next line it is suggested that the physician who was asked to perform the abortion be expected to exercise medical judgment as he would in the case of any elective surgery, where one seldom can provide exact guidelines. In reality I think what would happen is what happened in England. One has to face the fact that there are some doctors who would go into the abortion business for financial and other reasons. Some might feel this is a very important medical service to perform, and would go into it so the woman would not have to be faced with the problem of going to a doctor to see if she could convince him. She would know that there are certain doctors who did abortions fairly routinely. I think that is what would happen. It is not a pretty thing.

Dr. Ewalt: I do not see that abortion is a legal matter. It is hard for me to see that. I think it is like cosmetic surgery or sterilization surgery, a personal decision, and then finding the physician who would agree that it is warranted. To me the problem is that the patients, at least those whom we see, usually turn out not to want the abortion as much as they think they do when you first talk to them and then you find somebody's twisting their arm. We have a very limited sample and it is a very biased sample we see because we do not have anybody who does not have some sort of mental problem along with it.

I fail to see how the law can contribute significantly to this other than in the matter of right that people may have. The disturbing thing about it to me is that the fetus' rights are being grossly interfered with. To me that is the rather touchy point about all this. You might even find brothers and sisters urging an abortion if there is an estate to be shared with an unborn child. I do not know, maybe it is really a social decision and not an easy one to make. We tend to be very conservative here because in spite of these studies our experience has been—probably again because we have a very selected group of patients—that people do not always react as well to abortions as Simon's and some of these other studies would indicate.

Prof. Curran: I have been a consultant for a number of years for the University Hospital regarding abortions and I would say that that was their stand too. They are very conservative, but the psychiatric service was of the opinion that their experience with abortion was not very good. The women displayed a great deal of personal guilt later.

Dr. Stone: The anecdotal approach is unreliable. What we need are statistical studies. Stephen Fleck,[3] in an unpublished paper, pointed out that the incidence of postpartum psychotic states is about 1 per 1000. In contrast, when you look for postabortion psychosis, assuming that there are about 1 million criminal abortions a year, it turns out that the number is really almost undetectable.

Dr. Ewalt: I do not think that is the issue at all. I think the issue concerns patients who have had an abortion earlier and then later on find that they can not get pregnant. Or, who later on in life get depressed. It is true that these people look for something to castigate themselves with when they get depressed and if they have had an abortion that may be the item chosen. It has also been my experience that it is very difficult to get them to rationalize that as being a symptom and not a fact. They still carry this thing with them.

Prof. Curran: Have you found that any part of their guilt is the breaking of criminal law?

Dr. Ewalt: No. It is "I murdered my child."

Prof. Curran: Do you think if we removed law from this area it would have any effect at all?

Dr. Ewalt: No.

Prof. Curran: Do you think that it is "Well, the law says this is all right," and so she does not have as much guilt?

Dr. Ewalt: No. It is because it is an affront to their femininity, to their self-realization as a female.

Prof. Curran: Well, what if the laws say it is all right to do this? You have got a right to an abortion. Would that make the patient feel that there was not as much guilt?

Dr. Ewalt: I do no know. I think a woman who has had four or five children already and finds herself pregnant again, might take some solace in such a law. The really difficult case is the woman who has had an abortion and then finds later on that she cannot get pregnant.

Dr. Stone: Well, will you not agree that this is much more apt to occur if she has had a criminal abortion than if she has had a legal abortion in a hospital?

Dr. Ewalt: Oh, yes.

Dr. Stone: Well, I completely agree with you as to the psychodynamics of the guilt in that I do not think it would be affected by the criminal law. I think, however, that in considering the psychodynamics, the abortion itself is not as traumatic as the context in which it occurs. One must take into account the kind of humiliating circumstances that these girls have to go through to get a criminal abortion.

Dr. Ewalt: You misunderstand what I am saying. You see, I do not think the law has any role in abortion any more than in my decision to prescribe for a patient electric shock or psychoanalysis or some other treatment. The law protects the person's right that the practice be competent and proper or he can sue. This does not mean that I am in favor of wholesale or easily acquired abortions. I think the patient ought to have a series of interviews with her physician or that the situation be thoroughly explored that she does in fact *really* want the abortion. If that can be established, as far as I am concerned, the birth rate can drop ¾ and it would not bother me. I feel people make a lot of decisions that are more apparent than real and they do it all the time. They get talked into something that on second thought they really do not want to do. This is where I am hung up.

Dr. Greenblatt: The clarification of motivation can be a very tough and long job.

Prof. Curran: Are you suggesting that you go ahead with this long exploration of motivation? She would have the child by then.

Dr. Greenblatt: That is right. I think that here I am guided a little bit by what I read about the Peter Bent Brigham experience of trying to clarify the motivation of kidney donors. They found that you did not have to go all that deep, that most donors had pretty good reasons and they were thoroughly content with them. Then they followed them up and found that generally they were still pretty content with the contribution they made. They did not even feel that they needed psychiatric help in all instances.

Dr. Ewalt: I do not think they need psychiatric help in any instances in abortion, unless a patient is probably psychotic.

Dr. Greenblatt: I have been asked why the APA has not taken an official stand on whether psychiatrists should be involved in the issue of abortion. Well, the APA has studied this problem. I was on the council when it came up and the general attitude was to accept the ALI proposal.

Dr. Ewalt: I do not think you want to rule out psychiatric consultation because there are some people who are neurotic, some depressed, some psychotic, and some on drugs. With such patients I think the psychiatrist could help decide whether the woman might be ready to make a judgment. I refuse to see these kids who have had a misadventure and are a little upset about it. I will not give them slips for abortions. I do not think it is any of my business. It is not really a psychiatric reason.

Dr. Greenblatt: Back to the GAP report. Do you believe that leaving the decision to the woman primarily is a step forward?

Dr. Ewalt: I do not see how you can do otherwise. If you extend it to the father, I would say you should first extend it to the child. I find myself very ambivalent about this right of the unborn child.

Dr. Greenblatt: Since you, Alan, were one of the major architects of the GAP report does this satisfy you?

Dr. Stone: I agree with Dr. Ewalt in certain respects and disagree with him in others. I have no confidence that the medical establishment, in the way it is organized now, can provide this service equitably. That is, if it is a young girl who has had a misadventure and her father is Professor So-and-So of the medical school he may call up the psychiatrist and the psychiatrist may look into it, whereas if Miss So-and-So's father is a truck driver, he may say, "that's one of the misadventures of the young." It is not a psychiatric problem in that case. However, it becomes a psychiatric problem when it is his colleague's daughter. This is the kind of problems we get into.

We get into another kind of problem when the obstetrician does not want to have more than a certain number of abortions per month, especially if it is a hospital with an abortion committee and so forth. For example, he wants to do 30 abortions a month. If he is only going to do 30 per month, then there is a risk he is going to do them for his friends, or people who pay high fees. So, the problem remains: can one really hope and expect that the medical profession will provide abortions in an equitable manner? I have a real concern about that. I have a concern also even if the medical establishment does provide abortions equitably because I do feel differently than Jack in that if we were doing 3 million abortions per year in this country, I would be very upset by that fact. It says something about our values as a people and how we value even the potential for human life. It would suggest to me that as human beings we were in serious trouble.

There are also difficult problems from the perspective of social Darwinism as to what kind of women would decide to have abortions. We would be leaving it up to the women, which is understandable in terms of the legal point of view of rights. On the other hand, there is a strong possibility that the way abortions would be had would have profound social effects. If younger people have abortions and if a shift continues in that direction, then our population would change. The median age of the parent population would be going up. That would create certain kinds of changes in civilization as we now know it. I do not know how to cope with questions like these, I merely raise them. I think that some of the English have been very unhappy with the results they have had in terms of the average age of girls getting abortions in England: 17 or 18. I am told that is the majority in their group. They are concerned about abortion becoming the contraception of the young.

This leads to the larger question of the moral responsibility for intercourse, and the biological responsibility for intercourse. This troubles me. I can see the virtue in terms of correcting the injustices of the current system of such a proposal. I can also see such a proposal creating new kinds of problems, serious problems which I am concerned and worried about. I do not have Dr. Ewalt's confidence that the medical establishment can deal with the matters in a way that will be either equitable or will deal with the larger concerns.

Prof. Curran: How do you think that the Supreme Court would deal with the District of Columbia case, especially if by the time it gets there there may be another appointment?

Dr. Stone: You know, it is intriguing because the one thing that Father Drinan said is that he hopes the Griswold issue would not be used as the basis for dealing with abortion. I can not really second guess, but I think the argument of the American Civil Liberties Union, which I tried to make earlier, that the way the medical establishment is now functioning—the rich are able to get abortions and the poor are not—may play a part in the Court's decision.

Dr. Greenblatt: Is this true in England?

Dr. Stone: In England, it is possible to get an abortion on the National Health Service. Let me just say that there are sometimes so many delays in the National Health Service that many of the youngsters are forced to try and get enough money to do it privately in one of these clinics. In California, where they have a new liberalized law, they found that about half as many abortions were being done on people on California Medicaid as on private patients. That again suggests a certain inequity since it is probably true that poor patients really have as much need statistically for abortion as do private patients.

Dr. Greenblatt: I would like to hear how Bill feels on this issue.

Prof. Curran: Well, as far as this point is concerned, I agree with the basic principle of taking it out of criminal law. I think I share many of the ambivalences that Alan is expressing. My guess on the Supreme Court decision would be similar ambivalence and I think I would base this on a change in the Supreme Court in the decision written by Marshall on alcoholism. The Negro position on this one is that the objective of many of the people who want abortion is to abort the Negroes, with the idea that the poor should be rushed into these public hospitals and the poor should get abortions. I am not sure you will get the poor to necessarily agree that the Supreme Court and the Planned Parenthood League are right and we should abort the poor.

There will be ambivalence on the part of many of those justices about the problems of destroying the various kinds of rights in the child. I am inclined to agree with the Griswold decision which says, "remove legal constraints and allow people to make their own decisions." It may still mean that there can be various uses of law but in a way having to"make law" through the Supreme Court is a shame. Perhaps what you really want to do is take the law off completely for some years and see what happens, but give it a chance to come back in again if there are abuses. The Supreme Court could apply such a broad brush and outlaw all abortion laws. That could be a decision we could regret 5, 10, or 20 years from now, in which case the Supreme Court might have to reverse itself in a very difficult way.

Dr. Greenblatt: One final question. At this stage what it does is affirm the identity and individuality of the woman. Her individuality has been affirmed by the pill considerably. I think we see a change in the balance of male-female relationships. Will this do more in that direction? Will it create a much more emancipated woman? And what is it going to do to the total picture?

Dr. Stone: That is essentially a sociological question. I think in Japan it is quite clear that when abortion was readily available that it was part of a Japanese man's machismo to get his wife pregnant, and then for her to go and get a legal abortion and then he would get her pregnant again and then she would go and have another abortion because the good Japanese woman was not to interfere with her husband's esthetic satisfaction in sexual intercourse. That sociological reality of male dominance was not altered by the law but in fact it resulted in greater subjugation of women.

Psychiatrists will continue to recommend abortion without clinical basis because they feel that they are providing an important service to their patients. To say that psychiatry has no scientific basis for doing what it does for many of them, is extraordinarily troublesome if psychiatrists come at it from the individual clinical point of view. Some have suggested that it might help to get the law changed if all psychiatrists were to insist that there are no valid criteria to justify abortion, that abortion is a social responsibility. I am sure this would create a great public uproar, but whether it will help is another matter.

Dr. Greenblatt: Let me comment on that. As I say I was on the council when this issue came up and my council experience has taught me that it is not so much the nice pat bourgeois position of the psychiatrists. This issue was examined for its merits on broad intellectual grounds. The people on the council have a very objective view, or try to have one, of many things. The point was that the ALI proposal, which was brought to us a couple of years ago, looked like a big advance. So they felt they were taking a very useful position. What they do is they appoint a committee and this committee comes up with ideas which they affirm or not. They often have to judge whether taking a stand will do more harm than not taking a stand.

Now, a word might be said about GAP. The fact that GAP came this far is very interesting. I would think that this is the biggest step forward in the direction of white papers that GAP has taken for a long time.

Dr. Stone: I can tell you that the vast majority of GAP membership who voted supported this position.

Dr. Greenblatt: Let me say that any publication that goes to the member-ship gets a vast support, 70 per cent support, and you have to start at the 70 per cent base.

Dr. Stone: No. It was not just a vote on a report. We circulated a ques-tionnaire to the 180 or so members of GAP.

Dr. Greenblatt: Then this report is pretty much the consensus of the group. The fact that GAP has come out with something as controversial as this is a very bold step.

Dr. Stone: I would like to make a few more points in terms of the question you posed at the beginning, namely the rights of various people involved and responsibilities to the unborn child. There are several important questions about the state's rights. It seems to me that in a number of ways the state should have some rights. They might be counterbalanced by other rights, but the state might have some rights in terms of the general ethical values of society, the valuation that society places on life, the population changes, and so forth that I talked about earlier. There is also a responsibility with that right. If the state says a child has to be born, then the state has a respon-sibility to see that that child is taken care of properly. And this, it seems to me, has been sort of the major moral failing of the state. The state has insisted on children being born, but then has not really fulfilled its responsibilities to make sure that these children got the kind of adequate care in infancy which makes that life which has been guaranteed to them meaningful.

The thing that is important in this is that although one can say that the state has a right, there is no way that the state can confidently force a woman to give her child the kind of mothering it needs. If, as I think, the best data show that the increase in abortions is in the young—the 17 and 18-year olds—who do not want children, who do not want to raise them, who do not want that kind of responsibility, then I think the state cannot force those women to treat those children in the way they should be treated. Nor has the state provided the kind of institutional facilities which would take care of those children. Moreover, it has become more and more problematic during the last few years to get children adopted. Then if the state exercises a right in terms of demanding that the woman go to term what happens is that a lot of chil-dren are born who are not being taken care of and the state does not come forward to take care of them.

So much for the rights of the state and I emphasize those rights must be counterbalanced by responsibility. Similarly for the husband. He cannot force his wife to bring up the child properly. So if he insists on having the child and he is given the right, there should be a burden on him, just as on the state. Can he provide the quality of life that the child needs to develop in the way we feel children should be able to develop? That might be a test in some way of his rights in the hypothetical case I gave you. In all of these areas it seems to me the right is balanced off by responsibility and a lot can be gained from looking into how well people are prepared to fulfill that respon-sibility. If not, they just exert a right willfully and then the responsibility falls to the woman who did not want the child. So, it is on these kinds of considerations that one begins to say more and more, "yes, it's a terrible dilemma, there is no decent solution." But the least tragic seems to me to let the mother have the say. I would feel very unhappy if a law like this were not accompanied by a considerable effort introducing education about contraception and providing planned parenthood clinics throughout all sectors of our society and some effort to really cope through education with the ignorance that creates the need for abortion.

IN RETROSPECT

Note added in proof by Dr. Stone: During the past 5 years there has been what amounts to a revolution in the basic social, cultural, legal, and ethical values about abortion. This shift in values has occurred at such a rapid rate that the term revolution is not mere rhetoric. It is difficult to determine what has been responsible for this sudden transformation, but that it exists is evidenced by the rash of legislative action and judicial decisions, buttressed by the formation of voluntary groups supporting widesweeping change both in law and the provision of abortion services. The discussion which preceded occurred at a time when it seemed that change would come from the judiciary rather than from the state legislatures. Subsequent events in New York, Hawaii, and elsewere, dramatically altered this situation. If, for example, New York were not to enforce strict residency requirement, it is possible that many of the questions raised in this discussion—for example, the Supreme Court's reaction to the California decision—would become moot.

REFERENCES

1. American Law Institute: Model Penal Code: Proposed Official Draft, July 30, 1962, p. 189.

2. The Right to Abortion: A Psychiatric View. Formulated by the Committee on Psychiatry and Law, Group for the Advancement of Psychiatry, Vol. 7, No. 75, October 1969.

3. Fleck, Stephen: Some psychiatric aspects of abortion. Presented to the Connecticut Medical Society, May 2, 1968.

Legal Aspects of Abortion

By Samuel Polsky, LL.B., Ph.D.

THE MOST SERIOUS ADVOCATES of abortion reform would have agreed as recently as a few years ago that Western culture, steeped as it was in the traditions of the rights of the individual, would be most unlikely to alter the status of the fetus in a manner to permit abortion upon demand. But the indisputable fact, in 1970, is that the attitude toward abortion in the United States has entirely changed. No greater evidence is needed than the passage of an abortion on demand law, by the New York State legislature which only two years earlier rejected a far more limited attempt at liberalization of abortion. In a way, changes in attitude toward abortion are a mirror of broader changes in American society: rejection of authority for authority's sake and demand for increased personal liberties are paramount among the forces for change. Concern about the deleterious effects of over-population has induced a group as prestigious as the National Academy of Science to state that the community and society as a whole, and not only the parents, must have a say about the number of children a couple may have.[20]

Although such a viewpoint raises the very fundamental question of the extent to which society, as represented by a state, can intervene in the personal lives of individual citizens, while retaining the value of individual freedom, it is misleading to presume that society has been altogether silent on the issue of population control. The law in the United States has spoken to the issues of birth prevention, voluntary sterilization, and abortion, admittedly in an inconsistent and sometimes contradictory fashion. The question of the state's right to legislate with respect to birth prevention information and devices, at least with regard to married couples seeking birth control help, has presumably been laid to rest by the Supreme Court of the United States in the *Griswold* case.[5] It was held in that case that the Bill of Rights establishes a right of privacy, particularly applicable to the marital relationship, and that a Connecticut statute which made it a crime for any person to use any drug or article to prevent conception was unconstitutional in that it violates the right of marital privacy. The state may not impinge on the zone of privacy unless it can show countervailing and compelling state interests, and in the view of the court, there is no legitimate state interest in preventing unwanted pregnancies.

The law's stance with regard to unwanted fetuses is entirely another matter. Under most circumstances, it is a crime in every state in the union to terminate a pregnancy. Only danger to the life of the mother justifies the death of the fetus. In some states, substantial danger of grave impairment of the health of the mother is sufficient to justify an abortion;* in eleven states,† the law also

---

*Alabama, Arkansas, California, Colorado, D.C., Georgia, Kansas, Maryland, North Carolina, New Mexico, Oregon.

†Alabama, Arkansas, California, Colorado, Georgia, Kansas, Maryland, Mississippi, New Mexico, North Carolina, Oregon.

permits abortion if the pregnancy occurred as a result of rape or incest; and an additional justification for abortion occurs in nine of the states,* i.e., substantial danger of grave impairment or malformation in the fetus.

There is great pressure for reform of abortion laws, particularly in those states where the only justification for termination of a pregnancy is to preserve the life of the mother. To evaluate the forms which this pressure has taken and to propose a solution to the question of what the legal attitude toward abortion should be, this paper will undertake to analyze the policy behind current abortion laws, including those already reformed according to the pattern proposed by the American Law Institute.[8]

POLICY UNDERLYING RESTRICTED ABORTION

It is important to understand the policy behind prevailing abortion laws—not only because of the possibility that there is something worth retaining, but also to sharpen the justification for desired changes by direct confrontation with the policy that led to the old patterns. One compelling reason that abortion has universally been declared a crime in English and American jurisprudence, is society's recognition that a fetus is something more than an aggregation of cells in the mother's body. It is a very special aggregation with potential for independent life. Because preservation of human life is a fundamental value in our society, activities which tend to destroy human life are to be restricted. Destruction can be permitted only when other compelling values are threatened by the existence of that life. If one's life is imminently threatened, it is legal to use killing force to prevent it. That which would otherwise be murder is justified by self-defense.

Viewed in that light, it is easy to understand why abortion laws came into being and developed in the patterns that they did. When a fetus is in existence, a potential life other than that of the mother is at stake. If capable of human existence, it is an appropriate subject for legal protection, and the fact that laws regarding abortion exist at all reflects this.

This can be focused on by considering that laws on voluntary sterilization are rare indeed. Only three states—Connecticut, Kansas and Utah—provide criminal sanctions against sterilization. Many states provide for mandatory sterilization of mental defectives and these laws have withstood constitutional challenge,[2] as a valid exercise of the police power. Virginia[26] and North Carolina[11] have statutes which protect physicians from civil liability for damages resulting from non-negligent sterilization operations, if they perform the operation in a hospital on the basis of a written request of the patient and spouse, fully disclose the procedure and consequences, and wait for 30 days after receipt of the request to perform the surgery.

It seems, then, that except in those few states in which sterilization without medical necessity is a crime, the law is either indifferent to the fact of volun-

---

*Alabama, Arkansas, Colorado, Georgia, Kansas, Maryland, New Mexico, North Carolina, Oregon.

tary sterilization or actively encourages it by affirmatively protecting physicians engaged in sterilization activity, even though sterilization destroys potential human life as effective as does abortion. Opponents of birth control, of course, use this argument to assail permissiveness in this area, but birth prevention can be distinguished from both sterilization and abortion, not only on meta-physical grounds, but in a very pragmatic way. Birth prevention is a totally private act, and whether or not one can say that life prevention is life destruc-tion, no one other than the participants in the act of sexual intercourse is involved. On the other hand, both sterilization and abortion require the par-ticipation of at least a physician, and if permissible by law and therefore more freely available, hospitals and other medical institutions are involved. Because of this broader participation, society is already involved in the acts of steriliza-tion and abortion. The difference in the law's treatment then can be explained on the basis that there is a sensed difference between the potential for human life inherent in the reproductive organs of a man and woman and that of a fetus.

The relevant question is: when is the potential for human life sufficiently realized so as to be worthy of legal protection? In the case of sterilization, it would seem that society has made the judgment that as against the freedom of an individual to deal as he will with his own body, an unfertilized ovum or unfulfilled sperm is not sufficiently human to warrant the law's concern. At common law, abortion was an offense only if the pregnancy had continued to the stage of quickening.[16] Until the fetus had reached that stage of develop-ment, it was not, according to the majority view, sufficiently alive to be an object of the law's protection.* There are several plausible explanations for the choice of this stage of development as the dividing line between crime and noncrime. One is simply that during the development of the common law, reproduction was so enshrouded in mystery that no one could say with cer-tainty that a fetus was alive until its movements were perceptible to the moth-er. Only when there was certainty of life could an action hostile to that life be punishable as a crime. A court, speaking in 1923, implicitly accepts that as the reason for the "old" common law, acknowledges that now science is better, and suggests that the requirement of "quickening" can be explained as a prac-tical necessity:

> In a strictly scientific and physiological sense there is life in an embryo from the time of conception, and in such sense there is also life in the male and female ele-ments that unite to form the embryo. But law, for obvious reasons, cannot in its classification follow the latest or ultimate declarations of science. It must for purposes of practical efficiency proceed upon more everyday and popular conceptions, . . . That it should be less of an offense to destroy an embryo in a stage where human life in its common acceptance was not yet begun than to destroy a quick child, is a conclusion that commends itself to most men.[3]

---

* Several courts deemed the fetus to be alive from the moment of conception, but felt change should be made legislatively, not judicially. See: Mitchell v. Commonwealth, 78 Ky 204 (1879).

The common law did not long remain the law of the United States. In the nineteenth century, the state legislatures codified their criminal laws and often abolished the quickening requirement so that the fetus was protected from the moment of conception. It would be logical to presume that as legislatures considered statutes on abortion, they incorporated the more sophisicated scientific knowledge available at that time, recognized the potential for human life in the fetus at a time earlier than that of "quickening," and thus protected the fetus throughout the entire period of gestation. That this is a fair representation of what happened is asserted in a recent New Jersey case:

> The 1849 act and the subsequent legislative treatment reveal an unquestionable intention to enlarge the scope of the common law crime of abortion . . . The lawmakers were saying as a matter of public policy that the moment the womb becomes instinct with embryonic life, it should be unlawful to interrupt the ordinary development of that life "without lawful justification" . . . the most important consequence of the statute is the legislative recognition and sequential incorporation in the law of the principle that the child as a legal entity begins at conception; as of that time it has a legal existence as a separate entity, as distinguished from a mere part of its mother's body.[4]

If it is accepted that the thrust of the laws on abortion was to protect the life of the fetus, and that legislatures considered that life began at the moment of conception, it follows that the only permissible justification for termination of that life is to preserve the life of the mother. This is consistent with the bulk of our jurisprudence which permits acts which would otherwise be murder if they are for the purpose of self-defense.

But in attempting to evaluate the legislative intent behind the vast majority of abortion laws which permit termination of a pregnancy only if the life of the mother is endangered by the continuation of the gravid condition, evidence contradictory to that stated above cannot be ignored. In a careful study of the New York law concerning abortion,[7] documents contemporary with the passage of the law have been unearthed which indicate that the primary concern of the legislature was the health of the mother, and *not* the life of the fetus before the time of "quickening" was reached. In 1828, when the entire law of New York was undergoing codification, the Revisers proposed a law making it a misdemeanor to perform *any* surgical operation by which human life would be endangered, for example the amputation of a limb or cutting for a hernia, unless the surgery was necessary for the preservation of human life. At that time any surgery was fraught with risks because of the dangers of infection and shock. In the view of the Revisers, the danger was so substantial that the state's police powers, specifically that of preservation of the health of its citizens, permitted the state to abridge a citizen's liberty to risk his life in general surgery. An argument can be made from this that the legislative purpose in making abortion an offense from the time of conception was to protect the mother from the dangers of the surgery itself. This view is bolstered by the opinion of the New Jersey Supreme Court in its comments on the New Jersey abortion law passed only eleven years before the court spoke. That court asserts that the purpose of the New Jersey statute "was not to prevent the procuring of abortions, so much to guard the health and life of the mother against the consequences of such attempts."[17]

If this view is accepted as the policy behind the vast majority of state abortion laws, their constitutionality insofar as they restrict prequickening abortions is in serious question. Under its police powers, a state has vast power to restrict individual liberty. But a law fails as a violation of substantive due process if it is arbitrary or capricious, or the means selected by the law has no real or substantial relation to the object sought to be attained. If abortion operations are performed under conditions of asepsis, currently prevailing in hospitals, and occur in the early stages of pregnancy, the surgery presents virtually no danger to the health of the mother. Since the danger no longer exists, it can be argued that it is no longer legitimate for the state to restrict the pregnant woman's liberty to choose an abortion operation, at least in the first trimester of pregnancy. The alternate explanation of abortion law policy does not admit of constitutional attack on the grounds of due process. If the object of the state is to protect the life of the fetus, with that life defined as beginning at the moment of conception, it is a legitimate exercise of a state's police power to prohibit acts inimicable to fetal life even in the first trimester. Even presuming this policy base, abortion laws are vulnerable to attack on other constitutional grounds to be discussed later.

Whether the original intent of legislatures in extending the prohibition against abortion to the time of conception lay in its concern for the life of the fetus or in concern for the health of the mother is arguable and ultimately unanswerable. What is certain is the opinion of the American Law Institute that the main factor accounting for laws against abortion is ethical or religious objection.

> As the fetus develops to the point where it is recognizably human in form (4-6 weeks), or manifests life by movement perceptible to the mother ("quickening": 14-20 weeks), or becomes "viable" i.e., capable of surviving though born pre-maturely (24-28 weeks), it increasingly evokes in the greater portion of mankind a feeling of sympathy as with a fellow human being, so that its destruction comes to be regarded by many as morally equivalent to murder. Moreover, abortion is opposed by many on moral grounds not directly related to the homicidal aspects. For some it is a violation of the divine command to be fruitful, from which has been inferred also the sinfulness of homosexuality, contraception, masturbation, and in general all sexuality which is "unnatural" in the sense of not being procreative. Furthermore, legalizing abortion would be regarded by some as encouraging or condoning illicit intercourse, although this factor can hardly be a significant influence on the rate of illicit sexuality in a society where contraceptives offer reasonable assurance against need for the unpleasant and expensive prospect of abortion. Finally, discussion of abortion techniques, with its necessary reference to female sex organs, becomes for some a shocking violation of the conventions of communication to be dealt with as "obscenity."[9]

But even if thought to be immoral by a substantial number of state legislators, the question that must be faced is: should abortion be a crime? Our basic traditions demand that criminal punishment be reserved for behavior that falls below standards generally agreed to by the entire community. To use the criminal law against a substantial body of decent opinion would not only violate our notions of "ordered liberty," but would lead to widespread violation and sporadic enforcement. That a substantial body of decent opinion urging changes in abortion laws exists is not in question. Despite the current restrictions on abortions, it is estimated that there are one million illegal abortions a year in the United States,[6] and that they are in the main, sought by married women with several children, who for social and economic reasons feel that they cannot physically or financially care for another child.[18]

Faced with that fact, and the additional information that the abortion mortality rate in the United States is over 1 per cent as contrasted to 0.01 per cent in Russia where abortion is permitted and performed by physicians under asceptic hospital conditions, the American Law Institute undertook a study of abortion statutes as part of its effort to codify the criminal law. They based their solution on the following principles:

(A) Indiscriminate abortion must be adjudged a secular evil since the procedure involves some physical and psychic hazards.

(B) Abortion, at least in early pregnancy, and with consent of the persons affected, involves considerations so different from the killing of a living human being as to warrant consideration not only of the health of the mother, but also of certain extremely adverse social consequences to her or the child, e.g., bastardy resulting from rape; prospective gross physical or mental defect in the child.

(C) The criminal law in this area cannot undertake or proceed to draw the line where religion or morals would draw it.

(D) Criminal liabilities which experience shows to be unenforceable because of nullification by prosecutors or juries should be eliminated from the law.[9]

The salient portions of ALI Formulation are as follows:

(1) *Unjustified Abortion.* A person who purposely and unjustifiably terminates the pregnancy of another otherwise than be a live birth commits a felony of the third degree or, where the pregnancy has continued beyond the twenty-sixth week, a felony of the second degree.

(2) *Justifiable Abortion.* A licensed physician is justified in terminating a pregnancy if he believes there is substantial risk that the continuance of the pregnancy would gravely impair the physical or mental health of the mother or that the child would be born with grave physical or mental defect, or that the pregnancy resulted from rape, incest, or other felonious intercourse. All illicit intercourse with a girl below the age of 16 shall be deemed felonious for the purposes of this Subsection. Justifiable abortions shall be performed only in a licensed hospital except in cases of emergency when hospital facilities are unavailable.

(3) *Physicians; Certificates; Presumption from Non-Compliance.* No abortion shall be performed unless two physicians, one of whom may be the person performing the abortion, shall have certified in writing the circumstances which they believe to justify the abortion. Such certificate shall be submitted before the abortion to the hospital where it is to be performed and, in the case of abortion following felonious intercourse, to the prosecuting attorney or the police. Failure to comply with any of the requirements of this Subsection gives rise to a presumption that the abortion was unjustified.[10]

This formulation deserves evaluation because it is an attempt to mediate the rigid laws demanded by a moralistic view of abortion and also because it is influential on legislatures. It has already been adopted, with some changes, as the law in ten states.

Simply stated, the American Law Institute recommendation on abortion preserves the prevailing law in that it classifies purposeful termination of a pregnancy, at any state of gestation, as a felony. It does liberalize the permissible defenses to the crime. A physician may plead justification on the basis of his good faith belief that continuation of the pregnancy creates a substantial risk to the health of the mother, physical or mental. By explicitly incorporating the mental health justification, the ALI is recognizing that psychic justification is the most common ground for legal abortion in those states which permit abortion at all if continued pregnancy endangers the health of the mother.

It then proceeds from concern for the mother to professed concern for the potential child, and permits abortion if, again, in the good faith belief of the physician, there is substantial risk that the child will be born with a serious mental or physical defect. Reflection on this eugenic justification does not readily lead to the conclusion that concern for the child is the real policy behind its inclusion in the law. It is extraordinarily difficult to rationally take the position that the child would choose no life at all as against a defective life. It seems clear that the unarticulated policy behind the eugenic exception is concern for the emotional health of the mother who must bear such a child as well as the not insubstantial social costs of caring for a defective person.

The additional justification for termination of pregnancy recommended by the American Law Institute is in the event the pregnancy resulted from rape, incest, or illicit intercourse with a girl under the age of 16. Again, social considerations and concern for the mental health of the mother seem to lie at the core of this exception. Social and family disruption is great when a young unmarried girl bears a child. If the girl's family either cannot or will not care for the child, he becomes a burden on the state. And it does not take too much imagination to realize the stress that could exist in a family situation into which a child is born who was conceived in the course of rape or incest.

In recognizing situations other than preservation of the life of the mother which would justify termination of a pregnancy, the ALI pattern is an improvement on prevailing law. But it can be faulted on several grounds, the most fundamental of which is that the recommended statute is not consistent with the principles which it enunciates. The commentators purport to recognize that the criminal law cannot undertake to draw the line where religion or morals would draw it and, therefore, they consider some adverse social consequences: risk of defect in the child, bastardy because of rape. They say that they will not consider the fetus worthy of complete protection from the moment of conception, and yet fail to recognize that the adverse social consequences that the vast majority of women seeking abortions are concerned about is their financial and emotional inability to welcome another child into a family already large enough. If it is not concerned about morals, it would seem essential that the ALI confront the reason that most people wish to have abortions. If it is concerned about widespread violation of a law and sporadic enforcement, it must at least wonder about injecting another brand of morality into the subject: that is, the views of the ALI reporters as to what social consequences are adverse enough to justify abortion.

In addition to the fundamental flaw of illogic, there are two serious constitutional attacks to which even the ALI law is vulnerable. To fall within the limits of the fifth and fourteenth amendments "prohibition or denial of life, liberty or property without due process of law", a criminal statute must be precise. Its language must be such that the conduct prohibited by law is clear on its face. If one cannot determine the kind of activity declared to be criminal from the language of the statute or clear legislative intent, it fails by reason of vagueness. This argument has been accepted by both the Supreme Court of California[13] and a District Court of the District of Columbia[21] to invalidate non-ALI abortion laws.* The portion of the ALI law which permits abortion if the physician believes that there is substantial risk to the physical or mental health of the mother is equally subject to the attack. The problem lies in the statutorily undefined word "health." Individual physicians' perceptions of the degree to which a pregnancy must interfere with health to justify an abortion will necessarily vary. Many physicians undoubtedly subscribe to the World Health Organization definition of health: "a state of complete physical, mental and *social* well-being, not only the absence of illness and disease." Those who do, will in good faith believe that an abortion performed in the first trimester of the pregnancy of a married woman who already has five children and an income of $5000 per year, is legal. Upon his conviction for violation of the abortion statute, he will learn that health does not have that meaning, but what meaning it does have is uncertain. Most courts who have considered the question have rejected an interpretation requiring a showing of certainty of immediacy of death.[14] The District of Columbia court specifies the uncertainties inherent in their law which forbids abortions except "as necessary for the preservation of the mother's life or health."

> The word "health" is not defined and in fact remains so vague in its interpretation and the practice under the act that there is no indication whether it includes varying degrees of mental as well as physical health. While the law generally has been careful not to interfere with medical judgment of competent physicians in treatment of individual patients, the physician in this instance is placed in a particularly unconscionable position under the conflicting and inadequate interpretations of the D.C. abortion statute now prevailing. . . . There is no clear standard to guide either the doctor, the jury or the Court. No body of medical knowledge delineates what degree of mental or physical health or combination of the two is required to make an abortion conducted by a competent physician legal or illegal under the Code.[22]

The laws of New Jersey, Pennsylvania, and Louisiana are even more vulnerable to a vagueness attack, than those of other states. The Pennsylvania law,

---

*The California court in the case of *People v. Belous* reversed a lower court conviction of Dr. Leon Belous on the ground that a standard which permits abortion only when "necessary to preserve life" is so vague that it denies the accused of due process.

for example, simply says that anyone who has the intent to procure a miscarriage, *unlawfully,* uses any means to do so, is guilty of a felony.[12]

The last word has not yet been uttered in the "void for vagueness" controversy. The District of Columbia court invited direct appeal of its decision to the Supreme Court of the United States. It remains to be seen whether or not the Justice Department will decide to live with one District Court's opinion in the District of Columbia rather than risk attack on the predominant pattern of abortion laws throughout the country in the Supreme Court.

The second line of constitutional attack is based on considerations which the American Law Institute commentators completely ignore. Even in those states in which the only justification for abortion is preservation of life, legal abortion is frequently available to those women who can afford a psychiatric consultation which results in a certification that the woman is so distraught as a result of the pregnancy that suicide is predictable. In states which permit abortion because the pregnancy impairs the woman's health and under the ALI pattern, a psychiatric statement as to damage to mental health is even easier to obtain for those who are medically sophisticated and sufficiently affluent to pay private physicians for such consultations. It is the poor and uneducated who cannot through these means buy a legal, safe abortion performed under medical auspices, and who are reduced to the necessity of dangerous self-abortion or unclean, medically risky, illegal abortions. Poverty is a condition that administration of the criminal laws cannot hope to correct. On the other hand, when the administration of a criminal law has the effect of discriminating against the poor, there is a serious question of whether the law violates the fourteenth amendment mandate that a state may not deny to persons within its jurisdiction "the equal protection of the law." In practice, hospitals have been delegated the de facto responsibility of administering the states' abortion laws, and the practical determination of the legality of an abortion, because prosecuting attorneys simply do not question what goes on in the operating rooms of legitimate hospitals. The rules of most hospitals provide that the abortion committee decide on availability of an abortion based on the recommendations of one or two physicians. Those who can afford private physicians to press their case before the hospital committee are far more likely to obtain an abortion than those ward and clinic patients who rarely can approach the hospital house officers on the subject. That the state acquiesces in such a situation by failing to scrutinize the legality of hospital board decisions is state action and a classification in administration of a criminal law based only on differences in financial resources is invidious and a denial of equal protection of the laws.

Many would like to argue that a woman has a constitutionally protected right to choose whether or not she will bear a child which she has conceived, and therefore that any law abridging this right is a denial of liberty without due process of laws. They base this on language of the Griswold case indicating that there is a zone of privacy which the Bill of Rights protects which may not be impinged upon by state law. The ultimate source of this argument lies in the ninth amendment to the U.S. Constitution which provides

that "the enumeration in the Constitution, of certain rights, shall not be con-
strued to deny or disparage others retained by the people." In a decision of
March 5, 1970, a federal district court in Wisconsin accepted this reasoning
and declared the Wisconsin statute which prohibits abortion unless it is performed by a physician and is necessary to save the life of the mother to be
unconstitutional. The court said:

> An examination of recent Supreme Court pronouncements regarding the Ninth
> Amendment compels our conclusion that the state of Wisconsin may not . . . deprive
> a woman of her private decision whether to bear her unquickened child.
> The defendants urge that the state's interest in protecting the embryo is a suffi-
> cient basis to sustain the statute. Upon a balancing of the relevant interests, we
> hold that a woman's right to refuse to carry an embryo during the early months of
> pregnancy may not be invaded by the state without a more compelling public neces-
> sity than is reflected in the statute in question. When measured against the claimed
> "rights" of an embryo of four months or less, we hold the mother's right transcends
> that of such an embryo.
>
> • • •
>
> There are a number of situations in which there are especially forceful reasons
> to support a woman's desire to reject an embryo. These include a rubella or thalido-
> mide pregnancy and one stemming either from rape or incest. The instant statute
> does not distinguish these special cases, but in our opinion, *the state does not have a
> compelling interest even in the normal situation to require a woman to remain
> pregnant during the early months following her conception.*[1]

The Wisconsin court did not reach the question of the constitutionality of a
statute which makes termination of a pregnancy a crime after quickening of
the fetus. At that state of pregnancy, or more precisely, between 24 and 28
weeks of gestation, when a fetus is capable of sustaining life outside the
mother's body, it is certainly arguable that the state's compelling interest in
protecting a life is sufficient to transcend the woman's right to decide whether
to bear a child and to sustain the constitutionality of a statute making it a
crime to terminate a pregnancy afer that state of gestation has been reached.

The three constitutional arguments, "void for vagueness," denial of equal protection, and Ninth Amendment "right of privacy," do not completely obliterate
a state's right to regulate abortions under its police powers. Thus, it is permissible for a state to require that abortions be performed by qualified physicians, just as other acts which constitute the practice of medicine are required to be performed by licensed physicians under the state licensure laws.
And when the fetus is viable, when it is no longer capable of being considered
merely a part of the woman's body, it is probable that acts done for the purpose of terminating such a pregnancy may be constitutionally classified as
criminal. This is not meant to suggest that a state legislature must regulate
with regard to abortion. There are no constitutional strictures requiring that
a state regard any particular act as a crime, and where a criminal law of the
state embodies some morality which is not shared by a substantial body of
decent opinion, the better solution is for the state to have no law on the subject
at all.

Abortion reform has been a major concern of the state legislatures during the current legislative sessions, and three states have passed statutes which accept as a principle that abortion, at least in the early months of pregnancy, is a matter to be decided by a woman and her physician. Maryland's new law, which repeals its 1968 abortion statute based on the American Law Institute model, permits a licensed physician to perform a legal abortion in any licensed hospital in the state. A woman need not have been a resident of Maryland for any prescribed period before she may have an abortion, nor is the availability of abortion limited to the early months of pregnancy by law, although that may be so, as a practical, medical matter. This bill has been passed by both houses of the Maryland legislature, but has not yet been signed by the Governor. Hawaii's new abortion law is essentially the same as Maryland's, the major difference being that Hawaii requires that a woman have been a resident of Hawaii for 90 days prior to the abortion. The residency requirement effectively prevents women from going to Hawaii for the purpose of abortion and, in the judgement of the Hawaii legislature, protects the state from becoming an abortion mill. The New York law, which became effective July 1, 1970, permits an abortion to be performed for any reason until the twenty-fourth week of pregnancy. It must be performed by a licensed physician, but the law does not specify that abortions must be performed in a hospital setting. There is no residency requirement. After the twenty-fourth week of pregnancy, the only justification for termination of a pregnancy is to preserve the life of the mother.

State legislatures are going to be in the business of abortion reform for the foreseeable future, not only because of the pressure for liberalization, but also because of the likelihood that their existing statutes will succumb to some combination of constitutional attacks. If the recent enactments in Hawaii, Maryland, and New York are indicative of a trend, statutes which approach abortion "on demand" are predictable. A conjunction of two forces in contemporary American society make this prediction even more certain. One is the recognition that many of our most pressing current problems, the blight of the cities, increased incidence of crime, pollution of the environment, among others, are attributed to over-population. Some have compared current attempts at liberalization of abortion laws with the experience of Japan where in the 1930s, laws similar to the Model Penal Code were adopted. It was discovered there, as it is now recognized here, that the abortion problem was not solved by that sort of liberalization, and in 1948, abortion was legalized as a method of reducing the birth rate.[19] The second force which seems to be expanding at an exponential rate is the drive for women's rights. The thrust of this movement can be summarized by the words of Dr. Harold Rosen, long an advocate of abortion liberalization:

> Mature women, as mature human beings with all the respect and dignity to be accorded mature human beings, should have the right to decide whether or not they wish to carry a specific pregnancy to term. The responsibility for the decision, right or wrong, is already theirs. The extra-legal abortion rate shows that they have already illegally assumed it. *It should be theirs legally.*[15]

SUMMARY

Legal concensus would argue that abortion is not a private act of concern only to the parents, but involves the unborn child, the law, the medical profession and society. The ethical and religious morality which at one time lent support to antiabortion laws has since been replaced by a substantial body of public opinion highly in favor of the practice of abortion. Until abortion laws are rid of vagueness, no longer discriminate against the poor and the unsophisticated, and stipulate social indications for abortion as well as medical and psychological ones, they will continue to be inadequate to the needs and sentiment of the times.

REFERENCES

1. Babbitz v. McCann, U.S.D.C. E. Wise, March 5, 1970.

2. Buck v. Bell, 274 U.S. 201, 47 S. Ct. 584, 71 L. Ed 1000 (1927) In re Clayton, 120 Neb. 680, 234, N.W. 630 (1931).

3. Foster v. State, 182 WISC 298, 196 N.W. 233 (1923) at 301–302.

4. Gleitman v. Cosgrove, 277 A2 689 (1967); concurring opinion at 698.

5. Griswold v. Connecticut, 381 U.S. 479, 85 S. Ct. 1678 14 L. Ed 2 510 (1965).

6. Law, Morality and Abortion; Symposium: 22 Rutg L.R 415 (1968) at 420.

7. Means: The Law of New York concerning Abortion and the Status of the Foetus, 1664-1968: A Case of Cessation of Constitutionality, 14 N.Y.L.F. 411 (1968).

8. Model Penal Code 230.3(2) (Proposed Official Draft A62).

9. Model Penal Code, Tent. Draft No. 9, Comments 207.11 (1959).

10. Model Penal Code, Proposed Official Draft 230.3 (1962).

11. N.C. Gen. Stat. 90-271-275 (Supp. 1963).

12. Pa. Stat. Ann. 4718.

13. People v. Belous, 80 Cal. Rptr. 354 (1969).

14. People v. Abarbanel, 239 Cal App 2 31, 48 Cal Rptr. 336, State v. Dunkelbarger, 206 Iowa 971, 221 NW 592 (1928, State v. Hatch, 138 Minn. 317, 164 N.W. 1017 (1917).

15. Smith: (Ed.) Abortion and the Law, Western Reserve University Press 1967: Rosen, Psychiatric Implications of Abortion at p. 106.

16. Smith v. State, 33 Me 48 (1851); Commonwealth v. Bangs, 9 Mass. 386 (1812); State v. Cooper, 22 N.J. L. 52 (1849); Foster v. State, 182 WISC 298, 196 N.W. 233 (1923).

17. State v. Murphy, 27 N.J.L. 112 (Sup Ct 1858).

18. Taussig: Abortion, Spontaneous and Induced (1936) at 387-8.

19. Tietze: Induce Abortion and Sterilization as Methods of Fertility Control, Natl. Comm. on Maternal Health, Publication 27 (1965).

20. The Philadelphia Inquirer, Nov. 10, 1969, p. 11.

21. U.S. v. Vuitch, 305 F. Supp. 1032 (1969).

22. Va. Code Ann. 32-423-426 (Supp. 1962).

Abortion: The Catholic Viewpoint

By FRANK J. AYD, JR., M.D.

BEFORE CHRIST'S BIRTH the Greeks and the Romans built mighty empires. Each became as enamored of their successes, as modern man is of his. Each worshipped a human trinity of values—material possessions, power, and prestige. Each glorified beauty, high physical performance, and intelligence. Each engaged in wars, the savagery of which is comparable to what is happening on both sides of the war in Vietnam. Each exalted the "quality" of life and not the sanctity of life. Each dehumanized, perverted, and corrupted human beings by coercion or evil indoctrination. Much of their "progress" was founded on a neglect of or disregard of individuals' rights. As their affluence grew, there was a decay of appalling proportions in their moral values. Debaucheries and orgies became pervasive. The "inferior" were enslaved, banished, or exterminated. For unwanted children there were abortion and infanticide. The aged and the infirm often were murdered. There were those who praised and encouraged suicide as a noble act. And the Roman public was entertained by gladiators mauling and killing each other and by viewing the murder of thousands by animals. Thus to the Greeks and Romans human life per se was neither sacred nor inviolate and this attitude was prevalent when Christ was born.

In the pre-Christian era there were objectors to man's inhumanity to man. Hippocrates declared that physicians should not perform or enable a woman to procure an abortion. The Jews legislated against abortion and infanticide but the law was ignored by many. Then God became man. By this act alone Christ taught a new and revolutionary concept of man, his dignity and worth. Man, Christ said, is compounded of matter and spirit with a natural and a supernatural destiny. From his creator he has received life, the freedom to do good or evil, and the obligation of preserving his life and bodily integrity. Because man is the custodian and user, but not the owner, of his life and body, the uses he can make of these are limited and governed by divine law. Man was created by God for God. The State exists for the individual and not the individual for the State. This, of course, was contrary to what Aristole advocated in the interest of the State, namely that all babies beyond a legally defined quota should be sentenced to death by exposure. Although there is no record of Christ explicitly condemning abortion and infanticide, His followers did denounce these practices and as Christianity spread infanticide was abandoned and abortions waned.

For 2000 years the Catholic Church has denounced and opposed abortion. It will forever because it does not have the authority or the right to sanction the direct, deliberate termination of pregnancy whatever the state of embryonic or fetal development. The Church has consistently defended the right of the unborn to live. A careful perusal of the writings of theologians beginning with the early Fathers of the Church in the latter part of the

48

first century, the statements issued by the Councils of the Church, including Vatican Council II, and the pronouncements of the Popes, including Pope Paul VI, reveals an uninterrupted insistence that from the moment of conception life must be guarded with the greatest care and that direct abortion is morally wrong.

There are those who say that throughout its history the Catholic Church has changed several times its position on abortion. This is absolutely false. It has steadfastly held that human life begins with conception. It is true that over the centuries, as medical views on the viability of the fetus fluctuated, there have been different opinions not on the immorality of abortion but about the severity of the penalty or penalties to be applied to the person(s) responsible for the destruction of unborn human life. Since no one has ever known when ensoulment occurs, there have been varying opinions on this. There have been those who expounded the theory of successive animation of the human conceptus. They held that abortion of an unanimated embryo, although illicit, is not homicide; only the abortion of a fetus animated with a rational soul is homicide. But since the nineteenth century the official doctrine of the Church has been that ensoulment occurs at the moment of conception. Hence the Church in its legislation does not distinguish between a fetus with a rational soul and a living embryo, though not forbidding free scientific discussion of the question.

Admittedly the rational and prudent assumption that ensoulment occurs at conception may be proved false. Just as modern scientists have penetrated outer space, thereby acquiring new knowledge, by discerning for the first time what always has existed, so too are modern Catholic scholars acquiring new knowledge, making new discoveries, and evolving theological insights into heretofore hidden but eternally existing truths. If it should be discovered that ensoulment occurs some time after conception and the theory of successive animation proved, the voluntary, deliberate direct destruction of an embryo unanimated with a rational soul and of a fetus animated with a rational soul would be sins specifically distinct. But to the Church in both cases there certainly would be sin.

There are many reasons why the Catholic Church defends human progeny. It affirms the dignity of the human person, who is a creature of God and personally responsible to God. It upholds the value of existence for what it is in itself, for its worth in relation to sound judgement, moral conscience, civil society, the Church, and above all God. It proclaims that the right to live is an inherent prerogative of every innocent person, that is, of every person exempt from personal guilt and violation of order. Its viewpoint on abortion was expressed succinctly by Pope Pius XII, who said: "In what touches his being and essence, man has been created for God and not for anything created. . . . Now the child, even the unborn child, is a human being in the same degree and by the same title as its mother. Moreover, every human being, even the child in its mother's womb, receives its right to life *directly* from God, not from its parents, nor from any human society or authority. Therefore there is no man, no human authority, no science, no 'indication' whether medical, eugenical, social, economic or moral, that can show or give a valid juridical title for a deliberate and direct disposing of an innocent human life, that is to say, for an action which aims at its destruction, whether such destruction be intended as an end or as a means towards some other end which may itself be in no way illicit. Thus, for example, to save the life of the mother is a most noble end, but the direct killing of the child as a means to that end is not lawful. . . . The life of an innocent human being is inviolable, and any direct assault or aggression on it violates one of those fundamental laws without which it is impossible for human beings to live safely in society."

Abortion supporters contend that a fetus is not a human being. Some say it is merely a "blob of protoplasm," or, in the words of Dr. Alan Guttmacher,[1] a staunch abortion advocate, "nothing more than a potential human being." They seem oblivious to their own contradictions. If the fetus is not a human being, what is it that is damaged in the early weeks of its existence by viral infections such as rubella, and by drugs, chemicals, X rays, etc. which they say justifies abortion? If the fetus is not human, why are thousands of physicians and scientists spending millions of dollars and countless hours in research to develop a rubella vaccine? Physicians of all persuasions say it is unethical to test the recently developed rubella vaccine on women pregnant less than twelve weeks because of the risk that the vaccine may pass through the placental barrier and damage the embryo or fetus in the womb. If physicians did not consider an early conceptus human, they would not consider unethical the testing of the rubella vaccine in women in the first trimester of pregnancy. If the fetus is not human why all the scientific efforts to devise means of preventing birth defects, to fertilize ova outside the body in a test tube, to develop an artificial placenta, to determine the sex of a human embryo as early as possible, to chart fetal maturation until birth, to devise better technics of intrauterine transfusion, to perform surgery on the fetus in utero, and to administer drugs in utero, such as antibiotics, to stop infections before they do damage to fetal organs? If the fetus is not human, why are so many physicians and scientists advocating artificial insemination, genetic engineering, and genetic surgery to enable man to control the biological makeup of his near and remote descendants? If the fetus is not human, why does the U.S. Food and Drug Administration prohibit or caution against the administration of certain drugs during the first trimester of pregnancy? If the fetus is not human from the moment of conception, what is it and why must it be destroyed?

Regardless of how or when an abortion is performed, and there is no time limit on when a pregnancy can be terminated, what must be acknowledged is that the desired objective is the death of the living child in the womb to avoid the later threat of a living child outside the womb. Thus, abortion is not simply a method of birth control. It is a denial of the sanctity of life and an affirmation that the value of human life is not intrinsically determined. Those who advocate more liberal abortion laws are urging society to adopt a new social policy that determines who shall live. They proclaim that a woman has an inalienable right to destroy her unborn child, because she is the owner of her life and body and therefore can do as she wishes.

A moment's reflection on the implications of the argument that a woman is the owner of her life and body raises vital questions that cannot be disregarded. If this argument is valid, and abortion proponents categorically state that it is, then similar arguments also can be advanced by these people to justify suicide, euthanasia, mutilation of the body, submission to dangerous human experimentation, and other human actions that society now condemns. After all, if the law says I own my life and body, how can I be denied the right to be sterilized for contraceptive purposes, or the right to commit suicide and to request and have a merciful extermination when I decide my life is worthless?

There are individuals who contend that the Catholic Church by opposing abortion is forcing its beliefs on society. This is not true. The Catholic Church's teachings primarily are for its faithful, but it does have the grave responsibility by divine mandate to teach that all men have fundamental rights, one of which is the right to live. By defending the fetus' right to live, the Church is not only affirming the sanctity of human life but it is opposing the delegation to any individual the right to decide who shall live. By its insistence that innocent human life is inviolable, the Church is upholding one of the fundamental laws without which it is impossible for human beings to live safely in society. Furthermore, by its opposition to abortion the Church is being truly humanitarian. There is a contemporary trend to human degradation. Today many people believe that the "quality" of human life is more important than its presence, sacredness and inviolability. They assert that the quantity of people should be limited, especially those considered by them to be "inferior" or "unwanted" because of physical and/or mental handicaps or because they would be burdensome to others. Hence, they advocate contraception and sterilization to prevent the transmission of life, abortion or fetal euthanasia to destroy the unborn whose lives have been judged unworthy of preservation and protection, and voluntary euthanasia for the chronically ill whose lives have been declared useless.

Enactment of liberal abortion laws or the abolition of all laws governing abortion could be one of the worst possible social and moral calamities. As Dr. Irvine Page[2] aptly observed: "It is a lesson of history that when men become indifferent to death they become brutalized. This was the premonitory sign of the Nazi scourge and the same was true of Stalinist Russia. Life has a way of taking revenge on those who destroy it."

SUMMARY

The attitude that human life was neither sacred nor inviolate prevailed during the pre-Christian era when abortion and even infanticide were considered the usual methods of dealing with unwanted children. In the post-Christian era a new value was placed on the dignity of man and the worth of human life. For almost 2000 years the belief that human life comes from God at the time of conception, and that man is only the custodian of his life rather than the owner has underscored the Catholic Church's opposition to abortion by human interference. For the Church, abortion represents an act that denies the sanctity of life and assumes that the woman is the owner of her life and that of her unborn child.

Despite disagreement concerning the exact moment of ensoulment of the fetus and the argument that it is not human at all, the Catholic Church has never altered its position on abortion. However, it does not believe that it has forced its belief upon society. Rather, its position is to safeguard the fundamental right to live of all human beings.

REFERENCES

1. Guttmacher, A.: Indications for a Therapeutic Abortion. Debate filmed by Public Health Service (No. T-1720) National Medical Audiovisual Center, Station K, Atlanta.

2. Page, I.: What strange values. Modern Medicine, November 4, 1968, p. 65.

Abortion: The Mental Health Consequences of Unwantedness

By MILDRED B. BECK, M.S.W.

T HE CONSEQUENCES OF REQUESTS FOR INDUCED ABORTION, approved and denied, are the theme of this paper. A few preliminary observations may help to place abortion in perspective in the human life cycle.

To begin with, what is abortion properly for? If we identify the common goals of the antagonists and protagonists of abortion law reform or repeal, one actually is impressed with the degree and the extent of unanimity. Stripping away the rhetoric, there seems to be agreement on the facts that sexual satisfaction and reproduction are not synonymous; that responsible behavior —which precludes exploitation in human relationships, be it in the area of sexuality or any other interpersonal relationship—can be influenced to varying degrees by law, threat and punishment, but is never effectively controlled or regulated by external force. There also seems to be a rapprochement between the two opposing camps, namely, that pregnancy interruption is an important health and, often, lifesaving measure when there has been human or mechanical failure in preventing an unwanted conception. However, there is still a dichotomy between the unequivocal enunciation of philosophy and application of that philosophy in relation to abortion practices. For example, though many persons uphold the principle of the right to self-determination, this right is sharply restricted in relation to abortion for reasons that are primarily referable to sociopolitical considerations, the economic and social status of the woman requesting the abortion, the personal or religious convictions of physicians or abortion committee members—in short, the deciding factors have little to do with the abortion-seeking woman's needs or those of her unborn infant. Increasingly, support is given to the conviction that a given woman and her physician, taking into consideration all relevant circumstances, are the primary persons involved in the decision as to whether a particular pregnancy is to be interrupted.

If the foregoing is accepted as the major criterion, it may be desirable to add that abortion is *not* the method of choice for population control despite the knowledgeable assertion of distinguished demographers that worldwide induced abortion was and remains the major means of birth control. Actually, abortion is the only method of *birth control;* all contraceptive methods serve as means of *conception control*—an increasingly useful distinction. Abortion is *not* an effective means for regulating what some persons choose, quite erroneously, to refer to as the unprecedented increase in premarital heterosexuality.[24] It is *not* necessarily an act that contributes to, or subtracts from, moral or ethical values though it is often used in that fashion by some who espouse the rights of the embryo to the good life, but completely ignore the deeds that often condemn him after birth to an unspeakable fate. It is in this latter sphere that the epidemiologist proposes to throw some critically needed light.

Problems directly related to abortions have proliferated, and more myth than fact has been advanced to support dramatically opposing views. For example, it is asserted that women whose request for an abortion is approved, or denied, suffer varying degrees of guilt and depression; it is alleged that few women who threaten to commit suicide unless aborted actually do commit suicide; it is presumed that children born of unwanted pregnancies "generally become wanted after birth"; it is reported that unwanted babies can be placed readily in adoption or foster care, and so on. Systematic and hard evidence to support any of these pronouncements are simply nonexistent. Hence, we are again confronted with a major area for epidemiologic inquiry, namely, what happens in fact to the woman, the children, and the significant others in their lives when unwise, and frequently unjust, efforts are coercively made to influence human behavior.

History of U.S. Abortion Laws

It is important to draw attention to one additional bit of background information, the "life history" of abortion laws in this country. Incontrovertible evidence suggests that the early abortion statutes were designed primarily to preserve human life, to safeguard against human ignorance at a given point in time and place and to prevent the exploitation of the helpless by the powerful. Medical historians have shown that when the first abortion laws were placed on the American law books, any form of surgery, abortion included, was well-nigh a death warrant. To protect a woman from varying degrees of permanent invalidism, if not death, and to shield a family against the loss of wife and mother, abortions were wisely prohibited. Brilliant advances in knowledge and technology, however, have changed primitive and dangerous medical practices to highly sophisticated and safe procedures. In fact, Dr. Christopher Tietze,[34] Associate Medical Director of the Population Council, has recently observed that deaths due to induced abortions performed in hospitals have dropped to exceedingly low values in a number of Eastern European countries. He indicated that in the period 1957–1967, for example, only 69 women died among nearly 2½ million women in Czechoslovakia and Hungary—a mortality rate of 2.8 per 100,000 legal abortions. In the U.S., at least one eastern state where the recently revised abortion law has been in force for about a year, reports no deaths among that state's 2,134 legal in-hospital abortions during the first year.

If any "error" was committed by the pioneers who sponsored severely restrictive abortion laws, it was in their decision—or their acquiescence— to place these laws in the *criminal code* instead of in the medical practices or medical ethics codes where every other comparable law governing medical and surgical procedures is to be found. Despite the unjust and unwarrantedly severe penalties this has brought in its wake, it is conceivable that at the time the law was written, there may have been a compelling and defensible reason for surrounding it with the most stringent safeguards. Irrespective of the camp in which one finds oneself on the issue of abortion law reform or repeal, and notwithstanding the growing but tangible success of the "reformers" and the "repealers," it might be an important token of earnest to assume some responsibility for avoiding the "deceptions (inadvertent and otherwise) that must be spun not only in the commission of error but also in the retreat from it. . ."[8]

Although major changes in the law and medical and social practices are now underway and even accelerating, there still is dangerously little dependable data upon which to predict criteria for either wise action or desirable institutional programmatic changes. For example, existing abortion statutes are beginning to be struck down as unconstitutional because they are "too vague" in language to permit judicious and unequivocal interpretations, or they are found, in practice, to discriminate in favor of the privileged, the educated, and those who are majority group members. Perhaps the most important reasons for the findings of "unconstitutionality" of extant laws rests on the serious and damaging interference with the doctor-patient relationship and the infringements upon civil rights. The Supreme Court in California[21] and a Federal judge in Washington D.C.* have declared their respective laws invalid. The Massachusetts Supreme Court, at the time of this writing, is gathering testimony of experts on its abortion law and New York State is reportedly considering the timeliness of contesting the constitutionality of its severely restrictive abortion statute. Interestingly, the pressure to repeal American abortion laws follows upon the efforts, within the past three years, to liberalize state laws so that they conform to the recommendations of the American Law Institute embodied in their proposed Model Penal Code. The unanticipated reasons for disenchantment with the effects of the liberalized laws (of eleven states) are attributed to the fact that it has proved impossible in far too many instances to synchronize the administrative requirements of the law with the professionally indicated needs of women who seek abortions. This dilemma is compounded by the ambiguity of abortion laws and their infringement of human rights, as cited in the recent State Supreme Court decisions.

While the literature does not yet reflect the serious ways in which the administrative requirements of the liberalized laws often nullify, in actual practice, the intent of the recently "liberalized" laws, many grave problems are beginning to surface. For example, the safest, most expeditious and least traumatic pregnancy terminations are completed as *early* as possible in the first trimester. Persons closely engaged in the surveillance of the process entailed in shepherding a woman "through the administrative maze" have told the writer that there are distressing delays, after initial examination,

---

*District of Columbia, U.S. District Court Judge Gerhard A. Gesell, on 11/10/69, held the 1901 statute of the District of Columbia "unconstitutional" adding that any "competent licensed practitioner of medicine" may not be prosecuted for interrupting an unwanted pregnancy "at least in the early stages," for reasons satisfactory to himself and his patient.

in obtaining scarce psychiatric consultative time, in getting the latter's report out promptly, in presenting the case for decision to the abortion committee and, finally, in securing a hospital bed. A number of these steps could be obviated if, for example, *routine* psychiatric examinations were eliminated and if the patient and physician were permitted to decide whether it is essential or desirable for her to be aborted. One distinguished professor of gynecology and obstetrics, speaking in behalf of his colleagues, remarked with a note of irony, "we are entrusted with the task of wielding the curette but not with the necessary judgments to determine when it is indicated." He added that in no other surgical procedure is the physician's judgment routinely challenged. He offered no objection to psychiatric consultation to the surgeon who will perform the operation. Indeed, he welcomed it and pointed to its numerous potential advantages, as, for instance, the sharing of the psychiatrist's special insights so that they may be used in behalf of *all* of the physician's patients. An important secondary gain resulting from this practice would be to cement the bond between psychiatrist and surgeon rather than to undermine it.

A word of precaution appears essential to those who view either abortion law reform or abortion law repeal as the answer or even as an important solution to the public health and mental health implications of current abortion practices in this country. Legal changes, of themselves, do not create hospital beds or technical competence, nor do they insure wise decisions. They do not change firmly held attitudes—an important consideration among decision-makers—nor do they safeguard against as yet unwritten laws which may be as destructive, albeit in different ways, as the ones they replaced. These are, therefore, the added imperatives to seek firm knowledge about the import to public welfare of approved and denied abortions. The basic questions, namely, the relationship of antecedent history of abortion practices to present day needs, the complex factors that determine whether a woman will unswervingly seek an abortion, and the consequences of the ensuing socio-medical decisions are all interrelated and important not only to her and her family but to the total society as well.

The Outcome of Therapeutic Abortion

The search for hard outcome data has been a very unrewarding one.[1,5,9,11,15,17,22,26-28,32] Foremost is the fact that abortion until recently was essentially an illegal act no matter what the indications for it or by whom it was performed. Few people seem aware that large numbers of abortions have been performed by licensed, competent, and very often highly conscientious physicians, but under illegal circumstances. Funds for research, again as a result of the law, could not be made available. What little dependable data is extant is, therefore, of foreign origin. If American, the findings have been tucked away in obscure periodicals as part of other studies, or the cohorts are numerically small and without adequate controls or based on clinical hunches.

The most frequently cited work on the destiny of children is that of Forssman and Thuwe.[7] A brief summary from an annotated source follows:[10]

"The study deals with 120 children born after their mothers had had an application for legal abortion refused during the pregnancy. They were followed up to the age of 21, and their mental health, social adjustment and education level was compared with a control group of the first same-sexed children born in the same hospitals. 26.7% of the unwanted children were born out-of-wedlock against only 7.5% of the control children. The parents legitimized 5 of 32 unwanted children and 5 of 9 control children by marriage after childbirth. 60% of the unwanted and 28% of the control children were considered to have had an insecure childhood. The unwanted children were registered more often in psychiatric services and for antisocial and criminal conduct, and got public assistance more often than the control subjects. Fewer of them had pursued theoretical studies beyond what is required. They were more often exempted from military service. More of the females married early and had children early. The differences in these respects were often statistically significant but even if they were not, they indicated the handicapped position of the unwanted children in comparison to the control group. It is concluded that the very fact that a woman applies for legal abortion means that the prospective child runs a greater risk of having to surmount greater social and mental handicaps than its peers even if the grounds for the application are too slight to be accepted."

The Quality of Life of the Unwanted Child

The sources of the most important American data on the quality of life that confronts the salvaged but unwanted infant are the United States Children's Bureau and the Child Welfare League of America. They report:

> More than 300,000 children are now the wards of public and private agencies . . . upward of 100,000 are probably 'trapped' in foster care—have little or no hope of rejoining their parents— and are suffering severe personality damage as a result. Social workers call them 'the orphans of the living' . . . nearly half—46.5 per cent—of the children who are in foster care are placed because of parental neglect, abuse or exploitation. The rest? The reasons vary: broken homes, economic troubles, sickness, psychiatric problems. For one reason or another, the parents are unable or unwilling to care for their children. Mainly, foster children are rejected youngsters. And most show it.[13]

The existence of a link between the unwanted child and child abuse has yet to be clearly established through retrospective studies, but a few facts are important. From January through December of 1962, 662 cases of child abuse were reported[5] by all but two of the 50 states and the District of Columbia. They range in age from early infancy through 17 years, though more than half—55.7 per cent—were under four years of age. Of this group, one in four or a total of 178 succumbed to their injuries. Of the latter, 81 per cent were under four years of age and 53 per cent were under two years of age. It was found that fathers were responsible for 38 per cent of the total of 662 cases reported and were accountable for 22 per cent of the fatalities. Mothers, responsible for inflicting 28 per cent of the injuries, were also guilty of more serious injuries and 48.54 per cent of the fatalities. The remaining fatal injuries were inflicted by others who were entrusted with the children's care. While much of the onus for the serious crippling and deaths of children rests on child caretakers of all sorts, the awful truth is that "parents were responsible for 72 per cent of the injuries perpetrated on the 662 cases" and for "78 per cent of the total fatalities."[5]

To read about the types of injuries that these children are subjected to is harrowing. Moreover, few can afford to overlook the fact that reported cases do not by any means reflect accurately the number of actual cases of child battering. The psychologically abused child is even more difficult to count because the damage to him is not nearly so evident—unless and until he commits dramatically overt acts of violence himself thereby thrusting himself into public view. Under-reporting is, therefore, a serious problem that is yet to be dealt with adequately. Dr. James Brussel, the psychiatrist associated with the New York State Department of Mental Hygiene, recites the sordid day-by-day grim details of the meaning of unwantedness in the life of the man who has become publicly known as the Boston Strangler.[1]

A recent report[30] by Silver, Dublin and Lourie dealing with 34 cases of child abuse, concludes that the child who is subjected to violence in his early years shows considerable evidence of a predilection towards violence himself. It is important to ascertain how many of these children—possibly even how many of their parents—were wanted. We need to know how compulsory pregnancies reinforce latent tendencies, at least in some persons, toward aggressive and destructive behavior in the children who are born of these pregnancies.

There are important indirect sources of data, quite possibly suggestive of a relationship between "unwantedness" and schizophrenia. Kety points to the changing concept of etiology:[17] "the nurture-versus-nature controversy is becoming obsolete in the study of schizophrenia as it is in the rest of medicine. It is no longer a question of which is involved but how much, and the most important task appears to be the precise definition of the specific biological and psychosocial factors involved and the mechanisms by which they interact in the production and development of various forms of schizophrenic illness." Shakow,[28] in discussing the schizophrenic's failures in adaptation, observes that the "patient appears to . . . attain in his illness the satisfaction of early fundamental needs which, in contrast with normal persons, have never been adequately satisfied in the ordinary course of events, particularly in the familial setting. This 'ordinary course of events' includes the thousands, nay millions, of appropriate affective reinforcements of behaviors which over the years lay the ground for what we call normal development."

Goldfarb[11] reports on the detailed evaluation of the psychiatric status of the parents of schizophrenic children:

> In considering specific patterns of family organization which may be related to the ego deficits of schizophrenic children, we have noted clinically and confirmed by controlled and systematic study a paralysis of parental function in the families of many schizophrenic children. . . . This kind of parental atmosphere is characterized by extreme parental indecisiveness; a lack of parental spontaneity and of empathy with the child; an inability on the part of the parents to grasp their child's needs and to gratify them at a suitable time; and an unusual absence of decisiveness, control and authority. The extent of parental ambiguity and bewilderment is far beyond that noted in the ordinary life of families of normal children. Case studies have documented evidence of the pattern of parental perplexity, as defined, at the birth of the child or far before the parents recognized the deviance of their children.

> The 'perplexity' hypothesis and linked findings are significant in directing our attention to the deleterious impact on the developing schizophrenic child of an unpatterned climate which does not actively reinforce desirable traits and does not inhibit undesirable traits.

He advances one conclusion of special interest, namely:

> . . . there is consistent evidence that the families of 'non-organic' schizophrenic children are more deviant than families of 'organic' schizophrenic children . . . The families of 'non-organic' schizophrenic children are consistently aberrant.

It is desirable to draw attention to a few crucial issues raised by the foregoing accounts. The serious limitations of medical records as a dependable source of needed data was confirmed some time ago when, in a conversation with Dr. Goldfarb, the writer was told that the medical charts used by him did not reveal whether the pregnancy was wanted, whether the mother had or had not sought an abortion or had tried—and in what ways—to abort herself. The paucity of recorded information of this type is reiterated by other investigators. In a study of the hospital records of 230 nonwhite and 404 white mentally retarded children born in Baltimore during the period of 1935 to 1952, Pasamanick and Lilienfeld[20] found that "the complications of pregnancy appear to be related to mental defect in a way that is 'similar' to that of factors previously found to be associated with stillbirths, neonatal deaths, cerebral palsy, epilepsy, and childhood behavior disorders." They observed that "these and similar observations (suggest) the hypothesis of the continuum of reproductive casualty (which indicates an area within which lies the possibility of prevention of neuropsychiatric disorders). It indicates the need for extensive studies of the factors causing or associated with the complications of pregnancy and labor, since these not only influence maternal health and infant loss but apparently have an influence on the surviving infant."

This study, already 15 years old, raises the still unanswered question of to what extent in utero damage may be the result of poor or absent prenatal care or the determined effort of the woman to dislodge the conceptus.

Recent clues, according to a personal communication from Pasamanick to the writer, suggest additional facets of the overall problem that require study. As an illustration, he points to the very young female who, by virtue of youth alone, is already at great risk for complications of pregnancy and premature delivery. If one adds to this poverty, membership in minority groups and out-of-wedlock pregnancies, one finds other critical dimensions that must be taken into account by those concerned for the welfare of the mother and her infant. It may, therefore, be very productive to study the rates of pregnancy, in and out of wedlock, among the youngest age group and the rates of pregnancy complications and premature births as these may be related to psycho-medical morbidity in the mother and infant. It is, perhaps, possible that an important criterion for therapeutic abortions may emerge.

There are some ubiquitous and nagging queries that cannot be easily dismissed. "What kind of a mother can a woman make if the *rejection of the pregnancy is stable over time?*" "What kind of a mother does a woman make who threatens but does not complete a suicide attempt?" Is it defensible to maintain the position that the "responsible" woman will get an abortion if she really "needs" one; but the "irresponsible" woman will be forced to bear and rear a child? And how many of these "irresponsible" women—many of whom are alcoholics, mentally ill or retarded, or habitual drug users— are even aware that they have borne their third, fourth or eighth child, all of whom have already been farmed out after birth for placement? And what happens to these children? Moreover, what *really* happens over time to the woman who threatens suicide but does not follow through? How many of these are responsible for the cases of child abuse and infanticide previously referred to? How many go into severe postpartum depression with recurring depressions thereafter? The important point here is that, having decided that there is no immediate threat to the mother's life, an abortion is denied with no anticipation of the outcome or followup to support or challenge the correctness or the wisdom of decisions made. If no one follows these women to see what the consequences are to her health, mental health included, or if no one examines the quality of interaction that is possible between her and the totally dependent new infant, it becomes very much easier to *conjecture* about outcome. Unfortunately, the few studies we have on any of these issues are seriously deficient.

Caplan[3] reported on his experiences in Israel some years ago with a group of sixteen mothers, all of whom had several children and who were, in the main, warm and generous with their children *except* with the child in treatment. After many months of treatment, these tormented women finally disclosed the fact that they not only had strongly wanted to abort this particular child but had made numerous attempts to do so. The mothers' attitude that evidently emerged, in effect was: "From the moment of birth, the baby seemed to know what I had done to him. In fact, I think he may have been damaged somehow. Anyway, from the beginning he has rejected me— that is, refused to take the breast, to eat, to respond to any parental wish or requirement." These mothers, ranging from adequate to "good" with the patients' siblings, were otherwise inexplicably cruel and damaging to the patient.

Hendlin[14] in an intensive study of 25 male and female black patients in hospital following attempted suicide found special burdens attributable to American society's treatment of minority groups. But he refuses to "sacrifice psychology to polemics" and examines the colorblind common denominators in human anguish. He says:

> Many of the patients came alive only through acts or fantasies of violence. . . . The patients used a variety of devices to try to cope with their frustrations and rage. The suicide figures for young blacks would be even higher if they included those who literally and often purposely drank themselves to death. Most commonly, the origin of the patients' rage and violence was in maternal deprivation and cruelty. (One young woman said) 'My mother once told me she wished I

had been born dead or that she had gotten rid of me. The way things worked out, I wished it too. She kept telling me that when I was born everyone was getting rid of babies. She was never happy over anything I did.' . . . (Difficult though this patient's life was) it was no worse than that of the majority of the suicidal patients observed. In many cases, the mother had not raised the child herself but had given it to a relative when she was abandoned by the patient's father. Rage toward their mothers was the usual source of the violence expressed by so many. . . . From a psychosocial point of view, maternal deprivation is but a link in a chain, although naturally it is of primary imortance to the individual.

Wyatt[39] discusses women's positive and negative motives for having children from a psychoanalytic view. The spectrum of the healthy-unhealthy motives for child-bearing are impressively cited. He concludes, "the time has come to distinguish clearly *when* the reproduction of life adds to and continues man's well-being. . ." Surely we need to inquire into the circumstances when a mother and her future child are genuinely at risk, when intervention of a particular kind can resolve the problems that lead to the request for an abortion and when abortion is, or is not, the solution of choice. Not all women who request an abortion want one, and it is for this reason that, at present anyway, an especially heavy burden is placed on the doctor. For example, there is the woman who wants the child but is coerced by her partner, family or some other influential person to seek an abortion. There is also the woman who would quite willingly, perhaps, eagerly, come to term if she were given the specific service that she wants and needs. In Sweden, in contrast to our practice, a genuine effort is made to ascertain precisely what is wanted and needed before a decision is made.

Since we are primarily concerned in this paper with the relationship between unwanted pregnancies on the one hand and physical well-being and mental health on the other, we will refer only to two other areas that are in urgent need of examination. First, there are problems posed by the protagonists of the "rights and the dignity" of the unborn child insofar as they fail to state concomitantly what they perceive as their *obligations* to that child. It would seem a reasonable expectation that those who profess this attitude should, in addition, be prepared to distinguish satisfactorily between a *conceptus* that is still incapable of contributing independently to the sustenance of its own life *irrespective* of any and all available skill and resources at the command of science to keep it alive and, a *fetus* or "infant" who can be viably maintained in some fashion outside the uterus and independently of the biologic parent. In some respects, the law has more or less fixed this point. Most states permitting therapeutic abortions set the time limit up to the end of the first trimester. One state sets fourteen weeks as the outer limit, another sixteen weeks, two states permits it up to twenty weeks, one up to twenty-six weeks, and one up to "150 days." But beyond the first trimester, the states that have extended the time limit add qualifications such as that the outer time limit "applies only to rape or incest" or "only to preserve the women's life or where the fetus is dead" or "in cases of danger to life."[4]

This partial review of the plethora of literature that may be plumbed for clues to the meaning of compulsory pregnancies still leaves us with the methodological problem of how best to approach the enormously complex issue of "unwantedness" from the standpoint of its meaning to the person who is "unwanting" and the person who is the object of "unwantedness."

Many partial truths about the significance to women (and their menfolk) of pregnancy and childbearing were advanced, among others, by psychoanalysts two or more decades ago. Cumulative experience, together with the information yielded by prospective and retrospective crosscultural studies, have led to broader and deeper insights into human motives in reproduction.[39] It appears that some women *never* want to bear or raise children; some women *merely want to know* that they are capable of conceiving; some females, occasionally as young as 12, want "something to love of my own," not realizing at all that that "something" is in long and continuous need of being "refueled and drained" in addition to being unconditionally loved; some women want children, tragically and doubtless unconsciously, for abusive purposes; and some women want children eagerly and devotedly but "not *this* one" because of the serious probability of genetic damage, untoward family tragedy and the like.

The epidemiologist, possibly more insistently and tenaciously than others, emphasizes the singular importance of *asking the right questions,* and of the right persons. Epidemiologic methods of study are among the most successful in uncovering factors that are of etiologic significance. For the purpose of examining the natural development and course of physical and mental disorders in total populations, in identifying persons at risk and in tracing "outcome" as this relates to given forms of intervention, epidemiologically based research is strongly indicated. It appears of great importance to define "unwantedness" in measurable terms and its consequences for the "unwanting" person as well as for the person who is unwanted. Lawmakers, physicians, members of the mental health profession and social planners will all stand to profit from a better understanding of the overt and covert significance of unwantedness. Further, an epidemiologic handle on the problem of unwantedness in relation to the indications for abortion, may also yield a new and better way of dealing with the mental health implications of "unwantedness" as it concerns our programs for the aged, the mentally ill, the mentally retarded, the physically handicapped, the delinquent and all other special populations. In any case, there are few who would contest the premise that *all* children have the right to come into the world wanted and loved.[6] The human condition, without any particular assistance from us, furnishes all the slings and arrows that most mortals need or can cope with successfully.

SUMMARY

The consequences of abortion for the physical and mental well-being of the mother, the child, key family members and the community require investigation if judicious action is to accompany changing abortion statutes and practices. The literature to date, especially in the U.S., abounds in conjecture.

From the standpoint of an infant, there appears to be no positive relationship between a woman's biologic capacity to conceive and her ability to meet his physical and psychological needs. Hence, it is important to learn much more than we now understand about the life events that confront infants who are the products of enforced pregnancies. Important, too, is the significance to the mother and her family if she is compelled to bear an unwanted child.

REFERENCES

1. Brussel, J. A.: Casebook of a Crime Psychiatrist. New York: Bernard Geis Associates, 1968, p. 136.

2. Callahan, D.: Abortion: Law, Choice and Morality (in press).

3. Caplan, G.: The disturbance of mother-child relationship by unsuccessful attempts at abortion. Ment. Hyg. 38:67-80, 1954.

4. Checklist of Abortion Laws in the United States, Association for the Study of Abortion, N.Y.C. (Prepared by Roy Lucas, Director-General Counsel, the James Madison Constitutional Law Institute, New York, 1969.)

5. De Francis, V.: Child Abuse—Preview of a Nationwide Survey. American Humane Association, 1963. Paper presented to the 90th Annual Forum of the National Conference on Social Welfare.

6. Final Report of the Joint Commission on Mental Health of Children, Washington, D.C., Fall 1969.

7. Forssman, H., and Thuwe, I.: One hundred and twenty children born after application for therapeutic abortion refused. Acta Psychiat. Scand. 41:71, 1965.

8. Frankel, Max.: The Limits of Intervention. The New York Times Book Review Section, New York Times, November 16, 1969, p. 1.

9. Gebhard, P. H., Pomeroy, W. B., Martin, C. E., and Christenson, C. V.: Pregnancy, Birth and Abortion in the U.S. New York: Harper and Row, 1958.

10. afGeijerstam, G. K.: An Annotated Bibliography of Induced Abortion. Ann Arbor, Mich., Center for Population Planning, The University of Michigan, 1969.

11. Goldfarb, W.: Factors in the development of schizophrenic children: An approach to sub-classification. In Romano, J. D. (Ed.): The Origins of Schizophrenia. The Hague, Netherlands: Excerpta-Medica Foundation International Congress Series No. 151, 1967, p. 84.

12. The Right to Abortion: A Psychiatric View formulated by the Committee on Psychiatry and Law. Group for the Advancement of Psychiatry, Vol. 7, Oct. 1969.

13. Haitch, R.: Orphans of the Living: The Foster Care Crisis. Public Affairs Pamphlet No. 418, published in cooperation with the Child Welfare League of America, 1968, p. 203.

14. Hendlin, H.: Black Suicide. New York, Basic Books, 1969.

15. Jenkins, R. L.: The significance of maternal rejection of pregnancy for the future development of the child. In Rosen, H. (Ed.): Therapeutic Abortion. New York, Julian Press, 1954, pp. 269-275.

16. Kenyon, F. E.: Termination of pregnancy on psychiatric grounds: A comparative study of 61 cases. Brit. J. Med. Psychol. 42: 243, 1969.

17. Kety, S. S.: The relevance of biochemical studies to the etiology of schizophrenia. In Romano, J. D. (Ed.): The Origins of Schizophrenia. The Hague, Netherlands. Excerpta-Medical Foundation International Congress Series No. 151, 1967 p. 39.

18. Lieberman, E. J., and Swenson, D. D.: International Family Planning, 1966-1968. A Bibliography. National Institute of Mental Health, Public Health Service Publication No. 917, U.S. Government Printing Office.

19. Meyerowitz, S., and Romano, J.: Who may not have an abortion? JAMA 209:260–261, 1969.

20. Pasamanick, B., and Lilienfeld, A. M.: Association of maternal and fetal factors with development of mental deficiency. JAMA 159:155–160, 1955.

21. People vs. Belous, September 5, 1969. Supreme Court of the State of California.

22. Pohlman, E.: "Wanted" and "unwanted": toward less ambiguous definition. Eugen. Quart. 12: 19-27, 1965.

23. Rapoport, Judith: American abortion in Sweden. Arch. Gen. Psychiat. 13:24-33, 1965.

24. Reiss, I. L.: Premarital sexual standards. *In* Broderick, C. B. and Bernard, J. (Eds.): The Individual, Sex and Society. Baltimore, Md., The Johns Hopkins Press, 1969.

25. Richette, Lisa A.: The Throwaway Children. Philadelphia and New York, Lippincott, 1969.

26. Rosen, H. (Ed.): Therapeutic Abortion. New York, Julian Press, 1954.

27. Schwartz, R. A.: The role of family planning in the primary prevention of mental illness. Amer. J. Psychiat., 125:12, 1969.

28. Shakow, D.: Some psychophysiological aspects of schizophrenia. *In* Romano, J. D. (Ed.): The Origins of Schizophrenia. The Hague, Netherlands, Excerpta-Medica Foundation, International Congress Series No. 151, 1967, p. 65.

29. Shainess, Natalie: Abortion: social psychiatric and psychoanalytic perspectives. New York, 1968, p. 3070.

30. Silver, L. B., Dublin, C. C., and Lourie, R.: Does violence breed violence? contributions from a study of the child abuse syndrome. Amer. J. Psychiat. 126:3, 1969.

31. Simon, N. M., Senturia, A. G., and Rothman, D.: Psychiatric illness following therapeutic abortion. Amer. J. Psychiat. 124: 59-65, 1967.

32. Sloane, R. B.: The unwanted pregnancy. New Eng. J. Med. 280: 1206-1213, 1969.

33. Swischuk, L. E.: Spine and spinal cord trauma in the battered child syndrome. Radiology, 92: 733-739, 1969.

34. Tietze, C.: Personal communication.

35. Webber, R. L. Myths about birth control. Public Welfare. 27: 9-12, 1969.

36. Westoff, C. F., Moore, E. C., and Ryder, N. B.: The structure of attitudes toward abortion. Milbank Mem. Fund Quart. V. XLVII, Part 1, 1969.

37. Whitlock, F. A., and Edwards, J. E.: Pregnancy and attempted suicide. Comp. Psychiat. 9:1-12, 1968.

38. Winston, Ellen: A national policy on the family. Public Welfare. 27:54-58, 1969.

39. Wyatt, F.: Clinical notes on the motives of reproduction. J. Soc. Issues. 23: 29-56, 1967.

The Gynecologist and "Therapeutic" Abortion: The Changing Times

By Russell Ramon de Alvarez, M.D., and Martin B. Wingate, M.D.

M OST STUDENTS OF MEDICINE, at some time during their professional life—such as entrance into, or graduation from, some medical fraternity—express a portion of the Hippocratic oath, swearing that they will neither perform nor contribute to the procedure of abortion. Only few physicians who have any professional concern with pregnancy adhere to what they may have once sincerely stated, if not believed.

The definition of abortion is not uniform throughout the United States and varies in three particular respects: legal, statistical reporting, and medical (obstetric and gynecologic). In practically all states, abortion is a statutory crime consisting of the intent to procure an unlawful expulsion or removal of the fetus by artificial means, with or without the consent of the patient to the procedure. From the statistical point of view, most states do not require a certificate of live birth or of stillbirth if the pregnancy has not continued to the twentieth week of gestation or if the fetus weighs under 500 grams. Two states are exceptions to this rule. New York State requires a certificate of "birth" of all products of conception delivered regardless of the duration of pregnancy. The State of Pennsylvania requires that a stillborn certificate be filed for all pregnancies which terminate beyond the sixteenth week of gestation. The Committee on Terminology of the American College of Obstetricians and Gynecologists defines abortion as the expulsion or removal of all (complete) or any part (incomplete) of the placenta or membranes, with or without an abortus. The use of the terms "early abortion" and "late abortion" are not encouraged. Therapeutic abortion is defined as the interruption of a gestation before the twentieth week of pregnancy for legally acceptable, medically approved indications as treatment of diseased states. These terms largely designate those procedures designed to save the life or to preserve the health of the mother. Formerly, therapeutic abortions were justified only on the basis of a clearcut medical indication. Textbooks of obstetrics and gynecology written during the 100 years prior to 1965, considered abortion justifiable for such extremes as when a vaginal delivery of a viable child was impossible or when some pathologic problem incident to pregnancy threatened the life or the health of the mother. More recently emphasis has been placed on the conditions of the fetus which might terminate or endanger *its life.*

THE CHANGING TIMES AND NEW ATTITUDES

The gynecologist has always regarded himself as a physician first. His role as a physician is based upon a fundamental training, background, and experience dedicated to preserve the life and health of the pregnant patient and to preserve the life of the fetus. With all change there comes the paradoxical conflict of former education, experience, and background. As social circumstances change, so too do interpretations of existing education, practice, and law. The changing professional attitude regarding all population problems as they affect the gynecologist-obstetrician has probably emanated from social, economic, ecologic, political, geographical, and psychologic considerations. Now, new knowledge regarding the influence of relatively simple drugs on embryogenesis, and of relatively simple and subclinical diseases on the production of severe defects in the fetus, direct many gynecologists toward abortion as the only known method of preventing these defects.

Because knowledge brings with it change, and all change is dynamic, it is little wonder that any universal alteration in existing medical practice, legislation or moral code would be met initially by tremendous resistance. When, with great suddenness, the projected population "explosion" became reality to the entire world, organizations whose very names were formerly anathema, as well as medical practices and surgical procedures designed for limiting the population, soon became popular causes and topics which could be mentioned without fear at any level of society. Family planning, family education of ethical conduct, sex education, and an honest presentation of contraception, sterilization, and abortion are now matters presented to the public from a knowledgable medical source in terms understandable to the individual or group being taught.

Gynecologists as physicians, in the true sense of the word, are concerned with the humanitarian needs of the community. Most have, at some time in their professional life, prescribed medication for the prevention of pregnancy, performed surgical sterilization procedures, and terminated pregnancies with the primary objective of preserving the life or health of the patient. These same gynecologists have seen wholesale slaughter of young women by illegal professional abortionists, lay abortionists, and by patients themselves. The most common emergency seen in Departments of Obstetrics and Gynecology within the United States is induced, often infected, abortion.

THE ABORTION COMMITTEE

Every accredited hospital in the United States which permits abortion (and some which do not) have Therapeutic Abortion Committees. In the past, these committees, always made up of physicians, attempted to interpret the law. Even though the majority of the members of such committees had no idea of the ramifications of the enacted statutes, the meaning of consent, or even the definition of crime, many acted as judge and jury "to prevent the committing of a crime." The primary function of such a committee should be to judge the professional medical indications for abortion as well as to determine the merits of continuing or terminating the pregnancy. In this way the committee would review the procedural aspects and thus protect the safety of the hospital and the physician. The Therapeutic Abortion Committee at Temple University Hospital, for example, is a standing committee of the hospital and provides a mechanism whereby the hospital itself assumes the responsibility for reviewing the reasons for the abortion and permitting this to be carried out by its personnel and with hospital facilities.

If there is majority concurrence by the committee, approval for termination of pregnancy, prior to sixteen weeks duration of gestation, is granted. This is presumably to preserve the life or health of the mother, or for protection of the fetus arising from incest, rape, or conditions considered deforming (physical or mental) to the fetus. Once approval is granted in writing, the procedure may be carried out surgically in an operating room or by amniotic fluid exchange. Usually when the pregnancy has advanced beyond twelve weeks duration and the uterus palpable well above the level of the symphysis pubis, abortion may be negotiated by the intraamniotic exchange and installation of hypertonic agents. Where tubal sterilization also is requested, approved, and contemplated, abdominal hysterotomy and surgical tubal sterilization may be carried out simultaneously. The procedure is designated and promulgated as a therapeutic abortion and the removed fetal matter sent to the Department of Pathology and so recorded in the patient's hospital chart. A case summary of each therapeutic abortion records, among other details, the marital status, duration of separation if present, and the indications for termination.

THE GUISE OF "PSYCHIATRIC" INDICATIONS

The Pennsylvania law, as it relates to abortion, is recorded under the Penal Code, Section 718, and is summarized as follows:

"Whoever *unlawfully* uses any instrument or drug with intent to procure miscarriage commits a felony." This statute does not indicate the meaning of the word *unlawfully*. There probably have been no occasions for judicial examination of the significance of the use of the word "unlawfully" in the statute. Many of the crimes defined in the penal code are statutory expressions of what existed as common law. Under common law, abortion was permissible where it was necessary to save life; thus, it may well be that the use of the word "unlawfully" was originally meant to be equivalent to "without the necessity of saving life or preserving health." Preserving health may be viewed as a means toward saving life. The common law, as first written into a statutory code in Pennsylvania in 1860, undoubtedly originally implied this equivalence. During the past hundred years, with great improvements in diagnosis, prognosis and operative procedures it seems likely today that an abortion could be considered lawful if the alternative were the serious impairment of the patient's health, even up to the point of death.

Prior to 1965, justifiable indications for abortions were usually related to severely disabling physical disease such as heart disease, vascular disease, cancer, renal disease, massive deformity or severe respiratory disease. Relatively few abortions were carried out for emotional diseases and none for social reasons.

Nowadays, requests for therapeutic abortion are not truly therapeutic for the management of clearly demonstrated disease. While most of the requests for abortions currently referred to therapeutic abortion committees are allegedly

Table 1.–Summary of Therapeutic Abortions Performed at Temple University
Hospital for the Years 1965-1970 (Inclusive)

| | Indications for Termination of Pregnancy | | |
	Psychiatric	Medical	Total
1965	18 (75%)	6	24
1966	29 (85%)	5	34
1967	38 (88%)	5	43
1968	68 (94%)	4	72
1969	195 (95%)	9	204
1970 (6 mos.)	240 (99%)	2	242
Total	588 (95%)		619

psychiatric in nature, it is questionable whether these indications really present substantial risks to the physical or mental health of the mother. During the past year 95 per cent of the abortions carried out at Temple University were done for reasons suggested by psychiatrists, if not for psychiatric disease. Most frequently, referrals from psychiatrists request that consideration be given to therapeutic abortion because of the actual or implied threat of suicide or because of the presence of suicidal ideation. Since the law of Pennsylvania leaves a loophole whereby therapeutic abortion may be performed to save the life of the mother, the threat of suicide apparently qualifies as justification for abortion. Consequently, since no disease exists, it is difficult to justify the use of the term "therapeutic." In fact, it is our feeling that abortions are really being performed on demand and limited essentially by the number of hospital beds available for this purpose.

When no medical or gynecologic disease is present to justify therapeutic abortion, it seems wasteful and perfunctory indeed to assign the time and skill of two gynecologists and an internist to a committee to deliberate, assess, or even concur in the written suggestions and requests presented by one or two psychiatrists.

Physicians are faced with the dilemma of being involved in the practice of medicine in isolation on the one hand or looking at the entire picture of social reform, economics, ethics, education and public service on the other hand. The current trend of many therapeutic abortion committees in hospitals or of individuals or groups concerned with approving abortion requests is to try to justify abortion on purely medical grounds. This is very difficult to do in so many instances that there seems to be a tendency to interpret many patients' situation as disease where no disease actually exists. In our own hospital and its affiliated ones, it seems likely that most requests for abortion presented under the guise of a psychiatric indication are for some related social reason. These include such considerations as broken homes, the number of children adopted into or out of the home, the use of drugs by the individual pregnant patient concerned, alleged rape, illegitimacy, or simply the patient's statement of inability to cope with a child, whether wanted or unwanted.

The view and stand taken by the American College of Obstetricians and Gynecologists is liberal, certainly more liberal than some of the recently revised state laws. In May 1968, the Executive Board of the American

College of Obstetricians and Gynecologists stated that the College would not condone nor support the concept that an abortion be considered or performed for any unwanted pregnancy or as a means of population control. This group issued the following statement:

> Termination of pregnancy by therapeutic abortion is a medical procedure. It must be performed only in a hospital accredited by the Joint Commission on Accreditation of hospitals and by a licensed physician qualified to perform such operations.
>
> Therapeutic abortion is permitted only with the informed consent of the patient and her husband, or herself if unmarried or of her nearest relative if she is under the age of consent. No patient should be compelled to undergo, or a physician to perform, a therapeutic abortion if either has ethical, religious or any other objections to it.
>
> A consultative opinion must be obtained from at least two licensed physicians other than the one who is to perform the procedure. This opinion should state that the procedure is medically indicated. The consultants may act separately or as a special committee. One consultant should be a qualified obstetrician-gynecologist and one should have special competence in the medical area in which the medical indication for the procedure resides.
>
> Therapeutic abortion may be performed for the following established medical indications:
>
> 1. When continuation of the pregnancy may threaten the life of the woman or seriously impair her health. In determining whether or not there is such risk to health, account may be taken of the patient's total environment, actual or reasonably foreseeable.
>
> 2. When pregnancy has resulted from rape or incest: in this case the same medical criteria should be employed in the evaluation of the patient.
>
> 3. When continuation of the pregnancy is likely to result in the birth of a child with grave physical deformities or mental retardation.

It should be emphasized that the inherent risk of such an abortion is not fully appreciated by many in the medical profession and certainly not by the public at large. In countries where abortion may be obtained on demand (Japan, Soviet Union) the medical authorities indicate that the physical and psychologic sequelae following abortion still remain to be determined, to say nothing of the difficulty in ascertaining the mortality and morbidity rates where such practices are carried out. The general public in the United States does not realize that in those countries which permit abortion on demand, a large number are performed in physicians' offices, thus clouding the incidence of serious complications and even the contribution to an increased maternal mortality.

LEGAL VARIATIONS: GREAT BRITAIN

It is relevant to learn from the experience of others, and amongst the latest countries to liberalize the law on therapeutic abortion is the United Kingdom. This Act greatly liberalized the maternal indications. Risk, for example, to the physical and mental health of the pregnant woman or any of the existing children of her family, are grounds for therapeutic abortion and account can be taken of the pregnant woman's actual or reasonably foreseeable environment. Only two physicians and no Board is required, and if abortion is "immediately necessary" no consultation is necessary. Reporting of the abortion is mandatory and penalty set for a failure to do so. There is no specific mention of rape or incest in the Bill and there is a conscience clause to exclude physicians who feel unable to advise patients on religious or moral grounds. Part of the interest of this Act arose because of the failure in England of repeated attempts to revise its laws since the famous court decsion of *Rex v. Bourne* in 1938. The present law was, in fact, bitterly contested in the House of Commons for 27 continuous hours—the longest debate in the House for over 30 years.

In 1958 there were 1600 therapeutic abortions in England and Wales and 2800 in 1962. By the end of 1969 it is estimated that at least 35,000 therapeutic abortions will have been performed under the auspicies of the Abortion Act. Forty-five per cent of the women were married, the remainder comprising the single, widowed, divorced or separated; 2 per cent of the abortions were on girls under 16 and 14 per cent on girls aged between 16 and 19.[2]

It has become apparent that the Act was an imperfect piece of law-making. Although the purpose of the new law was to liberalize the indications for legal termination of pregnancy, it was nonetheless interpreted by the public at large as a fiat for abortion on demand, and many doctors are being pressured to accept this lay interpretation. Little provision was made to protect the patient from unskilled practitioners performing the termination of pregnancy, and no attempt made to make the public aware of the dangers and complications of the procedure.[1]

Death may occur from sepsis, hemorrhage, embolism, and renal failure; to judge from the Jugoslav statistics, a morbidity rate of not less than 5 per cent is likely. Perforation and scarring of the softened uterine wall is not uncommon and infertility, menstrual disturbance and chronic backache are often reported. Implantation endometriosis is noted with increasing frequency when hysterotomy has been employed to terminate the pregnancy.

According to some authorities many women, particularly married ones, are struck with remorse many years after the abortion, and prolonged depression is not uncommon frequently leading to the need for psychiatric treatment.[3]

Because a termination of pregnancy has a temporal urgency, the number of beds available to physicians for the treatment of other gynecologic conditions has been sharply reduced, and in Britain today women with such nonurgent conditions as uterine and vaginal prolapse may have to wait for surgery for as long as four years. The increase in the number of women seeking therapeutic abortion has also dramatically reduced the time available in office and hospital clinics for the investigation and treatment of benign and malignant disease, and it is common to have to deal with three or four requests for abortion each day. It takes longer to refuse a termination than to accede to one, and there is a tendency to take the line of least resistance.[3]

It has also become apparent that a working rule of "if in doubt, terminate," has been imposed on many physicians since a continued pregnancy might produce evidence which could form the basis of a civil action for negligence. The Act has also, as is so common with laws involving physicians, left the workings of the law together with its moral implications to the physician to interpret as best he may, and this, when coupled with public pressure, has left him in an unenviable position.[3]

A Word of Caution

It is obvious that in an increasingly permissive society, public pressure from social organizations will bring about changes in the statutes relating to abortion in most of the United States. Many physicans are of the opinion that some legal change toward a more liberal interpretation of the law on therapeutic abortion is in order, but it is only a vocal minority who are loud in their support of "abortion by demand." Those persons in the social pressure groups who are in the forefront of the cry for therapeutic abortion at the request of the patient alone might perhaps modify their demands if they were present, or indeed took part in the physical destruction of a fetus, which is a necessary step in any termination.

Many physicians in theoretical favor of a more liberal attitude to therapeutic abortion have become revulsed by its practical application to their practice. Their traditional training toward the preservation of life has not fitted them to accept its destruction with equanimity.

People behave irresponsibly if denied responsibility and the answer to "the abortion problem" is not the abortion itself but the prevention of an unwanted pregnancy. This can only be attained by a continuing effort to disseminate and apply information relating to birth control. Doctors, paramedical personnel and trained lay personnel have a vital role to play not only in giving contraceptive advice but in the whole field of health education.

Summary

Under the impetus of family planning and population control, many gynecologists who swore neither to perform nor contribute to abortion find themselves involved in the procedure. This provides a clearcut conflict in a person who is trained to preserve life but is asked to end it. On the other hand, physicians performing abortions do not wish to perform them for pseudomedical reasons. Therapeutic abortions for which there are no clearcut medical indications are performed under the guise of psychiatric ones when it is questionable whether there is any substantial risk to the physical or mental health of the mother. This suggests that abortions are actually being performed on demand, often for social reasons, and that abortion laws should be brought into line with the practice in many hospitals. Those who advocate abortion on demand might modify their demands if they were present, or indeed took part in the physical destruction of the fetus. The day of abortion on demand in the United States is already here, for example, the new legislation in Hawaii, Alaska and New York. Teaching hospitals in these states and even in states with laws, e.g., Pennsylvania, cannot continue to handle this new compression of hospital beds since the bed utilization is no longer available to patients with cancer, prolapse, pelvic infection and other gynecologic disease. Consequently, the teaching hospitals with high abortion inpatient census face a serious problem in recruiting residents, interns and students, to say nothing of qualified faculty. The most sensible policy to meet social needs as well as medical ethics would be proselytization of effective means of birth control.

REFERENCES

1. Editorial: Demand for abortion. Brit. Med. J. 1:5638, 1969.

2. Lewis, T. L. T.: The Abortion Act. Address to the Royal College of Obstetricians and Gynecologists and Churches Council on Healing, January 1969.

3. The abortion act in practice. Report on Symposium held at Royal College of obstetricians and gynecologists (England), Brit. Med. J. 1:5641, 136, 1969.

Psychological and Emotional Indications for Therapeutic Abortion

By Nathan M. Simon, M.D.

W HILE THERE HAS BEEN AN INCREASE in studies of the psychological and emotional indications for therapeutic abortion, the literature is relatively small and the quality of the studies markedly uneven. Problems in interpreting and comparing studies arise out of the varying size of the sample, differences in criteria for abortion, cultural and social differences between populations studied, lack of clarity in agreement about diagnostic terms and a relative paucity of firm measures which meet general acceptance. This last issue deserves clarification. Even those measures that have a wide range of acceptance may be too crude to provide adequate answers to questions that are remarkably complicated. Furthermore, information about number of hospitalizations, suicide attempts, additional pregnancies, etc., which was valuable initially to chart the outlines of what was terra incognita has become less useful as our understanding of the problem has enlarged. Data of that quality have not been easily applicable in predicting, with a high degree of accuracy, those specific women in which interruption of pregnancy would be therapeutic or harmful.

The Need for Clarification

The word "therapeutic" itself needs some definition as used in this context. Therapeutic for whom, is the question that needs to be asked. For the woman involved, her parents, her other children, her husband, the physician or the society in which she lives? Obviously there is an interaction here. What is therapeutic for one could be therapeutic for others but the possibility of the contrary situation also exists.

There is frequently an implicit, if not explicit, assumption that for an abortion to be "therapeutic" it must reverse or "cure" a long standing psychosis, neurosis or character disorder. Such assumptions are, to put it gently, unwarranted and unfair. Therapeutic here implies the maintenance of the optimal level of function of which the individual is capable, permitting her growth and maturation and the opportunity for an adaptive solution to a stress that is within her potential as well as the avoidance of unnecessary pain and suffering.

The term "psychological indications" in the title also deserves scrutiny. To some this phrase only refers to whether there is currently present or may occur in the future a major psychosis, serious neurosis or suicide. It has been used in contrast to the terms "social," "socioeconomic" or "humanitarian." The implication of this construction is that an event, such as an unwanted pregnancy in a woman in her forties or a birth to a 14-year-old unmarried girl, will have no psychological consequences of importance if it does not result in psychosis or suicide. The attempt to separate "social" and "humanitarian" from psychological is to imply that the social context and the events that occur within it do not significantly alter the psychology of the people who experience them.

"Psychological indications" has also been used in contrast to "medical indications," again as if to assume that women with medical problems exist in a nonpsychological world. For example, a 35-year-old woman with four young children and severe rheumatic valvular disease who very much desired interruption, was initially rejected as meeting the criteria for medical indications for therapeutic abortion, because the cardiologists felt confident they could keep her alive for the last six months of her pregnancy by confining her in bed in the hospital. The effects of six months of enforced bed rest in the hospital on the woman, her children and her husband were not considered as making a significant contribution to the "medical indications" for interruption.

The above illustrates the unreality of compartmentalizing indications for interruption of pregnancy. It seems almost a too obvious truism to state that the most valuable approach in considering a woman's wishes to interrupt a pregnancy would be to view the request in the broadest possible context. The need to compartmentalize indications for therapeutic abortion is an artificial device that has grown in part from the laws which regulate abortion in stringent and rigid ways and from a need for parties involved to avoid responsibility.

Discussion of therapeutic abortion is like discussion of other major social problems such as war, poverty, environmental contamination and population control, in that it is no longer just a matter of presenting facts for the purpose of instructing. Some facts at this point are well known. Some others may be years away from elucidation. In several Scandinavian countries, Eastern Europe, Japan, and England, changes in the law have made legal abortion readily available. It is possible that the liberalized laws may have caused changes, although the only identifiable changes to date are statistics like birth rates. The liberalized laws have not resulted in any increase in psychiatric illness in any of the localities in which they are in effect, nor have they produced any visible dissolution in the social structure of the countries involved. Therapeutic abortion today in the United States is still an adversary procedure. Open, honest, responsible, and intelligent medical judgment has been rendered virtually impossible in most parts of this country by restrictive legislation. Even where laws are not restrictive, prevailing attitudes of physicians often narrowly limit the application of the laws.[9,16,35]

THE SCIENTIFIC STUDY OF ABORTION

The data on the efficacy of therapeutic abortion which are currently available have been based on studies of: women after therapeutic abortion; women who requested therapeutic abortion and were refused; and, women who had obtained permission for therapeutic abortion but did not go through with the procedure. However, the data developed from these studies cannot be compared with ease. The problems introduced by interviewer-bias, differences in race, socioeconomic groups and social customs, the lack of universality of the procedure and the differences in diagnostic criteria or criteria for interruption, length of follow-up, etc., are easily identifiable obstacles.

The scientific study of therapeutic abortion did not begin until the fourth decade of this century when changes in laws regulating abortion in several European countries made it possible to examine large groups of women applying for interruption of pregnancy and to assess the outcome. Although Swiss and Scandinavian researchers produced the bulk of the early literature, in the last five years there have been reports from Eastern Europe, the United States, and England.

The Unwanted Pregnancy and the Unwanted Child

Central to the problem of therapeutic abortion is the problem of the unwanted pregnancy and the unwanted child. Ambivalence about pregnancy is a very common phenomenon. Even in women who have stable marriages and want additional children, there are periods during a pregnancy when negative thoughts about the pregnancy are quite conscious and where the wish not to be pregnant appears. For some women a specific pregnancy may be a complete catastrophe. For others all pregnancies may be. Studies of women who felt negatively enough about their pregnancy to apply for abortion and then were refused an abortion or did not go through with the abortion, can give some information on the outcome of these unwanted pregnancies.

Höök[13] studied 249 Swedish women 7½ to 11 years after they had been turned down for therapeutic abortion. Eleven per cent of these women had illegal abortions after their applications were refused, and another 3 per cent had spontaneous abortions. At the time of follow-up, Höök found that 53 per cent of the women had serious problems for several years after the pregnancy and finally "adjusted." There was another 24 per cent who *still* had pathological symptoms that were related to the pregnancy. Höök concluded that one-third of the women should have had abortions in order to avoid serious problems related to the pregnancy. What Höök does not explain is why the other 43 per cent who had serious and persistent problems should not have been aborted. Eighteen months after their applications were refused, 7 per cent of the women were unfit to work because of mental problems. In the period between eighteen months and the time of final follow-up an additional 13 per cent were unfit to work for the same reason. There was a difference between women with "deviating personalities"—psychiatric difficulties—prior to their application and women who were described as normal. There was 42 per cent poor adjustment in the group of women who had deviating personalities and 12 per cent poor adjustment in the women described as normal.

This data indicates the high price paid in persisting psychological problems by women who are judged to have deviating personalities prior to their pregnancy. However, a significant portion of normal women (12 per cent) also paid a high price in terms of poor psychological adjustment. Another fact of importance is the high percentage of women who sought and successfully obtained abortion in a subsequent pregnancy. In subsequent pregnancies 50 per cent of these women, even though they had been refused before, actively sought and obtained abortion.

Aren and Amark[5] followed 142 women who had permission to have legal abortions but chose not to have the procedure. Follow-ups were conducted three to five years later. Seventeen of the women refrained because sterilization was a necessary condition for the abortion. The authors felt that in 89 per cent the decision to have the child was justified, but in 11 per cent an abortion seemed indicated in retrospect.

A most important factor in this study and one that has been overlooked generally, is the fact that most of the women in this study voluntarily chose not to be aborted. Fifty per cent changed their minds regarding therapeutic abortion and another 25 per cent were persuaded (sic) by their gynecologists not to have the abortion. This group differs from the women studied by Höök. These women, while ambivalent about their pregnancies, still felt positively enough about them to turn down the abortion and go to term. This study when compared to Höök's emphasizes the importance of the woman's motivation. It should be added that in 57 women who became pregnant again in this series, only 42 per cent carried to term. The remaining 58 per cent had either legal, illegal or spontaneous abortions. This is far from a ringing endorsement for their prior decision to not go through with a legal abortion.

Sim,[32] an outspoken opponent of therapeutic abortion, has recently published some data which seems to support my interpretation of the Hook and Aren-Amark data. As far as can be interpreted from his writings, Sim has never recommended therapeutic abortion. He reported a series of 54 women of mixed diagnoses whom he had followed during pregnancy. This was a highly selected sample. These women, all married, were referred to him by general practitioners who knew of his interest in treating women with serious psychiatric illness during pregnancy. *Only four* of these women wanted to have their pregnancies terminated by a therapeutic abortion. That is, 93 per cent were apparently interested in continuing their pregnancy, while only 7 per cent wanted their pregnancies interrupted. One woman had recurring admissions to psychiatric hospitals following the pregnancy; another woman developed a puerperal psychosis. Sim does not indicate whether either of these women wanted to continue their pregnancy or wanted an abortion. Sim's data primarily indicates that in the group of women he studied, 93 per cent of whom did not want to be aborted, the pregnancy could be "managed" by a psychiatrist who never recommended interruption.

Granacher's[12] follow-up of 496 Swiss women refused abortion revealed that only 60 per cent of the married women and 43 per cent of the unmarried women had positive attitudes to their children. He also observed that the physical and mental development of the child was satisfactory in 78 per cent of the married mothers and 56 per cent in unmarried mothers. The differences between the groups increased with age.

Forssman and Thuwe[11] compared 120 children born after application for therapeutic abortion was refused, with another 120 children who were matched very carefully. The follow-up period was twenty-one years. The 120 children in the study group when compared to the control group, had more insecurity in their family life, higher psychiatric utilization, demonstrated more anti-social and criminal behavior, needed more public assistance, were more frequently exempted from military service, more frequently were underachievers as far as educational levels and married earlier. The authors concluded that children born under those circumstances run the risk of having greater social and mental handicaps than their peers.

There is other data of importance in the Forssman-Thuwe study not commented on by the authors. The original sample of women refused legal abortion was 196. Sixty-eight women, or 35 per cent, had some type of abortion, either spontaneous or illegal. One hundred and twenty-eight women went to term and produced a total of 134 children. Four of these children, (3 per cent) were stillborn; 8 died in the first year and another 2 before the third year of life. The infant mortality in the first year of life for this sample is 6.1 per cent. For all of Sweden in 1948 the first year infant mortality rate was 2.3 per cent. Since these were all unwanted pregnancies, one can wonder if the hostility engendered by lack of acceptance of the unwanted pregnancy is reflected not only in a high spontaneous abortion and illegal abortion rate, but also in the high rate of infant mortality.

The risks of unwanted pregnancy extend farther beyond the social and mental handicaps that Forssman alludes to. In 1966 there were 10,920 murders in the United States and one out of 22 of these were filicides.[14] Resnick,[30] in reviewing literature on child murders from 1751 to 1960 reported on 131 filicides in which the victim was one day old or older. The number of filicide-mothers was twice as great as filicide-fathers. Fourteen per cent were classified by Resnick as being motivated because the child was an "unwanted child," in 21 per cent the parent was acutely psychotic, in 38 per cent the filicide was associated with suicide, and 12 per cent were "accidental" and were usually the result of a fatal battered child syndrome. Twenty-seven per cent of the victims were under six months of age and 48 per cent under two years. In another paper, Resnick[31] reported on 37 neonaticides (the victim murdered in the first 24 hours of life by a parent). The murders were committed by mother in 34 cases. Of the maternal neonaticides 83 per cent were classified as being motivated because the child was unwanted and 11 per cent because the mothers had an acute psychosis. Their diagnoses are less frequently psychotic than filicide mothers. Illegitimacy is the most common reason given for neonaticides. Other reasons are extramarital paternity, rape, and seeing the child as an obstacle to parental ambition. One group of these women, described as extremely passive, exhibited pathological denial about the pregnancy. A second group described as having strong drives with little ethical restraints, sought and were denied abortion during the pregnancy.

Anthony's[3] report of group therapy of 12 mothers with murderous impulses to their children, suggests that even where the impulses are not acted on directly, the damage can be considerable. The children were in concomitant group therapy. Half the children were overtly disturbed; two severely so. Several of the children acted out the mother's wish by making suicidal gestures.

Vanden Bergh, et al.,[37] report data of a different type from a small group of women they studied who had undergone the Shirodkar operation (to correct apparent weakness of the musculature of the cervix uteri and prevent expulsion of the fetus before maturity). Nine women in their study were habitual aborters described as unconsciously unwilling to accept the feminine role as mothers and wives. The other nine women were a control group who had no history of habitual abortion, but who also had the Shirodkar procedure. All 18 of the women went to term after the procedure. In the study group 5 patients had postpartum psychosis and one of these subsequently committed suicide. Of the remaining four, three underwent psychotherapy during their pregnancy and were emotionally stable postpartum. In the control group one patient had a postpartum psychosis and none had psychotherapy during pregnancy. While the sample is small, the evidence is highly suggestive that unconsciously unwanted pregnancies in especially vulnerable women when allowed to go to term precipitate serious psychiatric illness.

Brew and Sidenberg[6] reported an incidence of 0.13 per cent psychosis associated with pregnancy and parturition in a large group of women in New York State. They also reported that psychoses associated with pregnancy accounted for 1.3 per cent of all admissions of women to psychiatric hospitals in New York over a 23-year period ending in 1946. Jansson,[15] reporting data from Goteborg, Sweden discovered 0.60 per cent of all parturient women exhibited "mental insufficiency" requiring hospitalization in a psychiatric hospital. Pugh, et al.,[29] in a review of female first admissions to mental hospitals in Massachusetts, indicate in the child-bearing age group a significantly higher than expected rate of women who were pregnant or recently delivered. These studies of large groups of women contain no information on how many of the women actually consciously wanted or did not want to be pregnant. Direct casual relationships cannot be deduced from such data, but they underline that pregnancy and parturition does not appear to be an innocuous state for some women.

THE RISK OF SUICIDE

Suicide and attempted suicide are risks associated with unwanted pregnancy. Whitlock and Edwards[40] have reviewed the literature on this subject thoroughly. They state, "suicide in pregnancy is not so uncommon as widely believed." The studies they mentioned in their excellent review of the literature have rates from 1-20 per cent for the incidence of pregnant women among all women who committed suicide. The incidence of pregnancy among women attempting suicide ran from about 6-12 per cent. Edwards and Whitlock's own study of attempted suicide of 483 women (Brisbane, Australia) showed a rate of 7.2 per cent pregnant women of all women under the age of 45. Whitlock and Edwards thought that about half of the 30 women's pregnancies were related to the suicide attempt. They also estimated that since 7 per cent of the women in the population are pregnant at a given time in Australia, the incidence of pregnant women in their sample then could be accounted for primarily as a matter of chance distribution.

In Höök's[13] material, 31 of the original 294 reported applicants reapplied for termination of pregnancy, for the same pregnancy, after they were initially refused. Twenty-four were approved. Of these, 14 had voiced serious suicidal threats to friends or members of their family. This would indicate that the Swedish Abortion Boards are sensitive to the threat of suicide and tend to be more responsive to those women whom they consider serious suicidal threats and, therefore, grant more of them permission for legal abortion. It means that the group of women who are not aborted have been culled for the most serious suicidal threats. Lindberg[20] came to a similar conclusion in his study. Therefore, it is not surprising that there are relatively few suicide attempts following refusal of an abortion application in Sweden. There were three suicide attempts in Höök's sample.

One thing frequently overlooked in evaluating women for termination, is that pregnancies themselves very often are suicidal or self-destructive gestures on the woman's part. In our own study[33] of 12 women who were aborted for medical indications, 11 knew about their illnesses before they became pregnant. They had been warned not to get pregnant and had been instructed about contraception. Many of these women were chronically depressed. Their pregnancies in the circumstances of their physical illnesses contained serious self-destructive elements. Even in those women who were not physically ill, pregnancies were often extraordinary exercises in masochism. Typical of this group is a 28-year-old, white, divorced woman, diagnosed borderline schizophrenic, with two latency aged sons. She permitted her exhusband to return to live with her episodically, even though he drank constantly and beat her frequently. She made no efforts at contraception, even though she knew a pregnancy would interfere with her efforts to support herself.

Granacher[12] thought that in four of the nine women (in a series of 496) who died following refusal of therapeutic abortion, the strain of pregnancy had a probable connection with death. It should also be clear that some women are behaving in a suicidal way when they expose themselves, often repeatedly, to the incompetents and frauds who perform many of the illegal abortions. Lindberg[20] found that in women who were likely to be deserted by their male partners, women with hysterical traits and those who made explicit threats about illegal abortion, the risk of "desperate" (i.e., illegal or dangerous self-induced) abortion was considerable.

Suicides and suicide attempts do occur in pregnant women, and, from Edwards and Whitlock's[40] work it appears that at least in half of the cases, the suicide or suicide attempt is related to the pregnancy. An impulsive suicide attempt in a pregnant woman is something difficult to guard against or prevent. The presence of serious suicidal thoughts and/or history of previous suicide attempts in a woman who has an unwanted pregnancy should put the psychiatrist on guard. Even Anderson[2] who is not a strong advocate of interruption emphasizes this and reports on a suicide who was turned down for therapeutic abortion.

The most important consequences of unwanted pregnancies are not reported in studies which analyze large groups of individuals. They are present in almost countless number in the anecdotal clinical literature. The suffering, pain and sorrow on the part of the mother, the child, the family and often the community in those situations in which the child is unwanted is documented with monotonous regularity in psychiatric case studies. This more subtle effect of the unwanted pregnancy and the unwanted child is the most difficult to demonstrate statistically but probably the most important.

STUDIES OF RESPONSES TO THERAPEUTIC ABORTION

Discussion of the literature on the efficacy of therapeutic abortion will separate the data into those that attempt to measure objective responses of women who have had therapeutic abortions and those that measure their subjective responses.

Although the data is scant, it is of value to examine the reports that have been made about the outcome of therapeutic abortion in women with certain psychiatric diagnoses. It must be acknowledged from the onset that comparisons are especially difficult because of the absence of shared diagnostic criteria and also because of differences in diagnostic terms used in the United States and Europe. In the literature, generally, there is a rather marked disinterest in making specific psychiatric diagnoses on the women studied. Several authors (Clark et al.,[8] McCoy,[23] and Jansson[15]) completely ignore the preabortion psychiatric diagnosis.

Ekblad's[10] series of 479 Swedish women who had therapeutic abortion is one of the richest sources of data relating to therapeutic abortion. These women were studied in a thorough and standardized way immediately postabortion and again 22 to 50 months after the abortion. Ekblad's paper is liberally laced with clinical summaries so the reader can draw his own conclusions from the material presented.

The psychiatric diagnoses of Ekblad's sample is seen in Table 1. A total of 18 women had been treated in psychiatric hospitals prior to the pregnancy for which they were aborted. Five of these women, all in the schizoid group, were diagnosed at follow-up as defectively healed schizophrenics. None of these women were actively psychotic at the time of pregnancy. The other 13 women were hospitalized for "reactive insufficiencies" and two of these had

Table 1.—Psychiatric Diagnoses of 479 Women Who Had Therapeutic Abortion (Adapted from Ekblad)

Psychiatric Diagnoses	Number	Per Cent
Normal	201	42%
Psychasthenic	91	19%
Anxiety and obsessive–compulsive states	81	17%
Dysphoric and depressive	21	4%
Sensitive	15	3%
Schizoid	19	4%
Explosive	20	4%
Hysterical	23	5%
Psycho-Infantile	8	2%
Total	479	100%

Table 2.—Self-Reproaches in 479 Women Who Had Therapeutic Abortion
(Adapted from Ekblad)

Response	Normal Personalities	Abnormal Personalities	Total
Satisfied	74%	59%	65%
Abortion unpleasant but no self-reproach	9%	10%	10%
Mild self-reproach	10%	16%	14%
Severe self-reproach	6%	15%	11%
Total	99%	100%	100%

been hospitalized for suicide attempts. A number of women diagnosed as "explosive," or anxiety and obsessive-compulsive, might be diagnosed as borderline schizophrenics in the United States.

Table 2 indicates the subjective responses of the women to the therapeutic abortion. It should be noted that self-reproach is *not* equated to psychiatric illness.

Ekblad's analysis of the women after abortion revealed that while 11 per cent of the total sample experienced severe self-reproaches, only 1 per cent of the sample (five women) were disturbed to the point where their capacity to work was impaired. All five of these women had long histories of neurotic illness prior to the therapeutic abortion (two were diagnosed as anxiety and obsessive-compulsive reactions; one anxiety neurosis; one dysphoric-depressive and one explosive). More significantly, Ekblad points out that in four of these women it was a break with their male partner that was related to the decompensation and not the therapeutic abortion. In the fifth woman, protracted difficulties with an alcoholic husband were more related to the later psychiatric difficulties than the therapeutic abortion. Therefore, in none of the 479 women was major psychiatric impairment after therapeutic abortion directly related to the therapeutic abortion. None of the 19 schizoid women in the sample, including the five diagnosed schizophrenics, showed marked psychiatric impairment related to the therapeutic abortion.

Ekblad found only one variable significantly related to the development of self-reproaches post-therapeutic abortion. That variable was whether the woman had been influenced by others to have the therapeutic abortion (Table 3). Clearly those women who are persuaded by others to have an abortion are the greatest risks to develop self-reproaches after abortion.

Table 3.—Self-Reproaches for Therapeutic Abortions among Women Who Had Been Influenced by Others to Apply for Legal Abortion (Adapted from Ekblad)

	Total No. = N	Self-Reproaches No. = n	n as % of N
Psychically Normal			
Influenced by Others	9	4	(44)
Not Influenced by Others	192	29	15
Psychically Abnormal			
Influenced by Others	19	15	(79)
Not Influenced by Others	259	72	28

Ekblad's clinical vignettes indicate over and over again situations in which the women either appear to be operating at a stabilized level following therapeutic abortion, or show signs of improved functioning. His findings emphasize again how important the women's wishes are in determining the outcome of therapeutic abortion. It is clear that even very sick women, who on their own reach a decision to terminate a pregnancy, do very well following interruption of the pregnancy. None of the 18 women who were hospitalized prior to the therapeutic abortion for psychiatric illness were hospitalized after the therapeutic abortion for psychiatric illness during the follow-up period. One woman was hospitalized for a suicide attempt made after her lover abandoned her.

Our own series[33] had seven women (15%) diagnosed as schizophrenic in a total of 46 women who were aborted for a variety of indications. There were another seven (15%) with neurotic depression, 15 (33%) with personality trait disturbances, and 17 (37%) with no diagnosis. Of the seven women diagnosed schizophrenic, most of whom were borderline at the time of the abortion, two had subsequent psychiatric hospitalizations but neither of these hospitalizations were connected with the abortion. One woman with a diagnosis of neurotic depression had a hospitalization subsequent to the therapeutic abortion, again this was not associated with the therapeutic abortion. Two women with personality trait disturbances had psychiatric hospitalizations unrelated to the therapeutic abortion and one woman with a mild personality trait disturbance had a severe depressive reaction requiring hospitalization immediately after the therapeutic abortion. This woman was ambivalent about the abortion and was pressured into it primarily by her physician. This woman was aborted for a medical illness (multiple sclerosis).

There were five women who had psychiatric hospitalizations prior to their therapeutic abortions (three schizophrenic reactions, one agitated depression, and one personality trait disturbance). In three of these, their psychiatric condition was improved after the abortion (one agitated depression and two personality trait disturbances), and the remaining two (schizophrenic) remained unchanged.

There were two other important findings in this study: The first is that sterilization is often more of a problem than the therapeutic abortion itself. Significantly more women in the study who were sterilized had problems with guilt after the abortion. This agreed with the findings of McCoy[23] but not with Ekblad.[10] It is also in agreement with Aren and Amark's[5] findings that 17 women of their sample turned down an opportunity to have a therapeutic abortion because sterilization was insisted on as a condition to the abortion; second, the women who presented themselves for abortion were a selected lot in terms of their psychodynamics. These women as a group had demonstrated significant difficulties in their identification as women, especially the biological aspects of femininity and major conflicts about dealing with sadomasochistic impulses with great tendencies to acting out these conflicts.

Peck and Marcus's[27] series (of 50 women) revealed 36 per cent of the women diagnosed as schizophrenic, 18 per cent diagnosed depressed, 16 per cent with personality trait disturbances, 6 per cent with anxiety reactions, and 24 per cent with no diagnoses made. Only one patient, a woman aborted for first trimester rubella, was worse after the therapeutic abortion. This woman had deep religious convictions and had been forced into the therapeutic abortion by her husband. Peck rated 68 per cent of the 25 women who were aborted for psychiatric indications as having improved, in terms of their psychiatric illness, following the therapeutic abortion. He rated 20 per cent of the women who were aborted for nonpsychiatric reasons as improved psychiatrically following the therapeutic abortion. Twenty-four of the 25 women aborted for psychiatric reasons consciously did not want to be pregnant and all 25 strongly desired interruption of the pregnancy. Peck also comments on finding much masochism present in the group of women he studied, both the psychiatric and nonpsychiatric indications group.

Patt et al.[26] studied 36 women all aborted for psychiatric reasons. Nine (25%) were diagnosed as psychotic (the suggestion is that most of the women were schizophrenic), 14 (39%) borderline, and 12 (33%) as neurotic. There is no breakdown of the results by diagnoses. However, in the six-month period immediately following the abortion, 20 women showed prompt remission of psychiatric symptoms that had appeared with pregnancy. Of 15 women who continued to have psychiatric symptoms for up to six months, in 50 per cent of the cases the symptoms represented continuation of pre-existing severe mental illness. The long-term outcome for these women indicated that 26 women (75%) were improved following therapeutic abortion; 4 women (11%) were unchanged, and 5 women (14%) appeared to be worse. Two of these women related their worsened condition to the therapeutic abortion and the other three did not. Eight women reported that the abortion experience led to emotional growth and maturation. Patt et al.[26] make two other interesting observations: First, even though some women claim to have consciously manipulated the evaluation interview, these claims appeared to be an effort to deny severe mental illness. That is, these women could not admit to themselves that they were as sick as they really were at the time of the abortion. They were actually sicker than they claimed to be retrospectively; second, three women in this series concealed serious suicidal ideas at the time of their psychiatric evaluation. These women appeared to be inviting the psychiatrist to turn them down so that they might be "justified" in making a suicidal attempt.

Levene and Rigney[19] studied a sample of 76 women of whom 21 per cent were diagnosed as schizophrenic, borderline or schizoid (only one was overtly psychotic at the time of evaluation), 36 per cent hysterics, 14 per cent depressive reactions, and the other 29 per cent personality trait disturbances or no diagnosis was made. The one overtly schizophrenic woman in this study was still overtly psychotic after the abortion. The sample as a whole showed a marked lifting of depression in the six-month follow-up period. Only 14 per cent reported any increase in depressive symptoms but none of these 14 per cent related their increase in symptoms to the abortion. Levene found the women in his sample had many conflicts with sadomasochism and a high incidence of hysterical diagnoses.

There are only two studies in the literature whose findings are at variance with the above. Malmfors[21] (Sweden) reported about 12 per cent of her sample had suffered impairment of mental health following therapeutic abortion. All had various neurotic complaints before the abortion. The design and execution of Malmfors' study and her interpretation of her data have been seriously criticized. Malmfors' diagnostic criteria are vague, and she does not distinguish between guilt and psychiatric illness. Furthermore, there is little information about pre- and posttherapeutic abortion, psychiatric illness and incapacity, and the interviews were all done in the homes of the subjects.

Aren[4] (Sweden) studied 248 women. He found that 23 had severe guilt with symptoms such as insomnia, decreased work capacity, nervousness, which were common in that group. Unfortunately, Aren does not distinguish between guilt and psychiatric illness and Aren also makes no reference to the preabortion psychiatric evaluation of the women in the study.

Jansson[15] found that 1.9 per cent of the group of 1773 women who had undergone legal abortions in Goteborg developed psychiatric illness which required hospitalization following the abortion over a four-year period. In half of those women the hospitalization was unrelated to the abortion. Women in Sweden who have therapeutic abortions are a high risk group. They are selected primarily on the presence of psychiatric difficulties, although the legal indications, i.e., humanitarian, socioeconomic, etc., tend to mask this. Ekblad,[10] Jansson,[15] and Simon[33] all are in agreement that women with serious psychiatric difficulties prior to abortion, are more liable to have serious psychiatric difficulties after abortion. They point out that this does not indicate the abortion stands in a causal relationship to the postabortion psychiatric problems. These findings in women who have undergone therapeutic abortion are very similar to the findings of Höök,[13] and Aren and Amark,[5] who found that among women who had been either refused therapeutic abortion or did not go through with therapeutic abortion, those with more psychiatric pathology prior to their pregnancy also showed more pathology subsequent to carrying the pregnancy to term. In every study the overwhelming majority of women who evidenced serious diagnosable psychiatric illness prior to abortion remained stable or improved after therapeutic abortion.

Most studies of subjective responses of women with therapeutic abortion are in good agreement. Niswander,[25] Levene,[19] and Peck[27] (United States) all report better than 95 per cent of the patients they sampled were pleased with their decision to have a therapeutic abortion and felt the therapeutic abortion was the best answer in the situation they were in. Patt[26] (United States) reported 90 per cent of 35 women positive about the procedure, and Clark, et al.,[8] (England), found that 90 per cent of 120 women were wholeheartedly satisfied with the outcome of the therapeutic abortion and another 2½ per cent were acquiescent and only 2½ per cent were dissatisfied. Mehlen[24]

(Germany) found that 90 per cent of a group of 243 women thought the legal abortion was the best solution to their problems and only 10 per cent regretted their decision to have the abortion. Twenty per cent of a group of 100 women studied by Aren[4] in Sweden indicated they were dissatisfied with the therapeutic abortion and would not undergo therapeutic abortion again even though there were another pregnancy. No data on subjective responses to therapeutic abortion are available from eastern Europe where the numbers of procedures are in the hundreds of thousands per year.[36]

INTERPRETATION

The data reviewed above has been much belabored recently to "prove" a variety of points. There are some findings which seem to lend themselves to a single interpretation rather than multiple interpretations. First among these is that a woman's conscious motivation to terminate a pregnancy is of overriding importance in evaluating whether an interruption will be therapeutic. Second, psychiatric diagnosis as such, seems to be of less importance. Women who have severe psychiatric illnesses prior to their pregnancies and abortions clearly are at greater risk following the abortion. But these women are a greater risk even without abortion. The overwhelming majority of women from all diagnostic groups do well following abortion and respond to abortion as a positive therapeutic event. Third, unwanted pregnancies are not innocuous events and have pathological effects on the mother and the child. Fourth, suicidal thoughts in pregnant women who have unwanted pregnancies cannot be summarily dismissed as unimportant. In addition, the manner in which some women seek illegal abortion can be best understood as suicidal or self-mutilative behavior.

SPECIFIC INDICATIONS FOR THERAPEUTIC ABORTION

An understanding of the above factors provides a beginning for a rational approach to the psychological indications for termination of pregnancies. The prime indication is a deep-seated conviction on the part of the mother that the pregnancy is unwanted and she does not want to carry it to term. It is an evaluation of this conviction that is of primary importance. Whether its source be psychotic delusions that the fetus is destroying her from within, feelings of overwhelming helplessness and shame arising from her social situation, or murderous impulses directed toward the fetus or the father, is of less importance than the presence of the conviction itself and of the salient place which it occupies in a woman's mind.

Early interruption of a pregnancy appears therapeutic in cases where there is evidence of serious preoccupation with suicide or where suicidal thoughts are present in impulsive acting out hysterical women and of course, where the woman wishes interruption. Interruption of pregnancy appears specifically therapeutic for a depression that is initiated by an unwanted pregnancy[19,27] and which may persist long after the child is born if interruption is not utilized.

Therapeutic abortion should be considered in a woman with a history of postpartum psychosis. Women with one postpartum psychosis are a high risk group for the development of another postpartum psychosis. Over 40 per cent of the women studied by Protheroe[28] who had a puerperal psychosis and became pregnant again developed another psychosis. Twenty per cent of Martin's[22] series had another puerperal psychosis.

In the process of evaluating a woman for interruption of pregnancy, where psychosis or severe neurosis is present, where suicide is a possibility or there has been a history of a previous postpartum psychosis, the most critical issue is not a specific psychiatric diagnosis but rather how the woman is responding to the pregnancy. Sudden onset of depressive symptoms, suicidal preoccupation, depressed mood, agitation, anxiety, sleep and appetite disturbances, confusion, etc., the appearance of or increase in bizarre behavior (psychotic thinking, delusions, hallucinations, inappropriate affect) statements relating to hating the baby or the father of the baby, references to aggressive threats to the baby, bizarre statements about self-induced abortion, are all ominous signs which need be seriously considered. Another extremely important factor is the presence of marked denial of pregnancy. Especially in women pregnant out of wedlock, denial of and/or delayed recognition of pregnancy is an indication of serious pathological response.[31] In addition, evidence that indicates loss or threatened loss of an important figure who is related to in a markedly ambivalent way is also important.[10] A careful assessment must be made of the manner in which the pregnant woman is currently dealing with and has in the past dealt with rage and destructive impulses. History of poor control of rage and/or brutal behavior toward children on the part of the woman (and of the woman's parents, since mothers who brutally attack their children have often been brutally treated by their own parents) may be of help in assessing a likelihood of problems developing with aggressive impulses during the puerperium.

There are four other specific areas in which psychiatric indication for abortion can be stated with some clarity: incest; pregnancy in women who have been raped or who because of subnormal intelligence or extreme youth, do not understand the consequences of the sexual act that led to the pregnancy; pregnancy in the presence of severe physical illness; and the possibility of serious congenital or hereditary defects in the child.

Although there are no specific studies of the effects of incestuous pregnancies on the women who carry to term, I have not been able to discover any scientific voices raised in support of encouraging maintenance of pregnancies from incestuous unions. The genetic data on incest of first-degree relations are quite striking. In two recent studies[1,7] less than 50 per cent of the offspring of first-degree incestuous matings were normal. In addition to numerous congenital anomalies in the offspring, 40 per cent of the offsprings were mentally retarded. So it is clear that the genetic outcome is depressing in such unions.

First-degree incest is of two rather distinct types: parent-child, and between siblings. In parent-child (almost always father-daughter), the daughters tend to be somewhat older than in sibling unions. Also, the psychopathology is much more overt and serious in nature (with psychosis very frequently present). There is also the greater likelihood that the father and/or daughter will be subnormal intellectually. Brother and sister partners usually demonstrate less serious pathology, are much more likely to be of normal intelligence, and tend to be younger. The effects of carrying a pregnancy which resulted from incest to term cannot be separated from the effects of the incestuous union itself. Certainly the far graver situation is the father-daughter union as far as pathogenic effects are concerned. Actually, few of these situations present themselves for consideration of abortion since the pathology in such families usually tends to support the incest. It is only when there is some disruption in the pathological family equilibrium that psychiatrists or welfare agencies are involved. In any case, where such women do present themselves, leaving the dismal genetic outcome aside, there are clearly good reasons to recommend interruption. The psychiatric literature is replete with case reports detailing the pathogenic effects of incest, especially father-daughter incest and particularly incest that occurs in adolescence and adulthood.[17,34,38]

There is no study comparing the outcome in raped women who carry pregnancies to term and those who do not. Again, the situation literally speaks for itself. The burden rests clearly on those who would claim that carrying such a pregnancy to term would do no harm to the woman (and her family). Those who would not recommend interruption of a pregnancy due to rape, must provide an adequate answer to the woman who would be forced into carrying a pregnancy to term that was forced upon her.

Pregnancy of a severely mentally retarded woman whose level of functioning would make it impossible for her to care for the child presents another situation in which interruption is justified. In milder cases of mental subnormality, the recommendation should revolve around the women's wishes and the degree of acceptance of the pregnancy. Although there are some suggestions that offspring of mentally subnormal parents have a higher risk of being subnormal themselves, this cannot be the prime reason for the interruption and must be secondary to the consideration of the woman's psychological responses during the pregnancy.

The problems relating to pregnancy in adolescents are complex. To point out that child bearing begins at 13 or 14 in some primitive cultures, as one author has done recently, is not exactly relevant to the emotional stresses an adolescent will face in the United States when she becomes pregnant. I do not wish to oversimplify or attribute causality where only relationships are present, but the following seem relevant. Most early adolescents are singularly unprepared psychologically to assume the functions of caring for and raising a child and almost none of them do. Out of wedlock children of white adolescent girls are almost invariably placed for adoption. Out of wedlock children of black adolescent girls are almost invariably cared for by the girls' mother or mother surrogate. In Waters'[39] series only 10 per cent of the girls (who were nearly all black) returned to school. He saw the pregnancies in these girls as a critical point in the development of the "symptom of failure" which characterizes their later lives. Where care is assigned to others one can justly question the purpose of the pregnancy—was it punitive, or due to disinterest or neglect, or because of racial prejudice and stereotype (i.e., it is all right for Negro adolescents to have babies out of wedlock), or to provide fodder for the adoption industry. Well over one-half of all teenage marriages are pre-cipitated by pregnancy. Failure rates in teenage marriages are much higher than marriages contracted by older partners.

There are some situations in which a pregnancy originally desired, or at least felt to be tolerable, becomes unwanted. Rubella infection in the first and second trimester is the most common situation in which this occurs. Some women are seriously stressed and adversely affected when faced with a high risk of severe uncorrectable pathology in a child. These women desire and elect interruption when it is available. Our series[33] and Peck's[27] revealed these women respond very well to therapeutic abortion. Those who are committed to bearing a baby usually become pregnant again quickly. Sophisticated genetic diagnostic techniques in early pregnancy also make it possible to avoid the anguish that dominates women who live with the knowledge that their children run a risk of serious hereditary illness.

Pregnancy in the face of severe physical illness in the pregnant woman requires careful evaluation of what the effects will be of treating the illness to preserve the pregnancy. Some women will find such treatment more stressful and damaging than therapeutic abortion. This is especially true where the treatment requires lengthy hospitalization, bed rest and other limitations of physical activities that keep them from caring for their families or going about their usual activities. The other element that must be considered in women with serious physical illness is a careful estimation of the suicidal intent in-volved in the woman's pregnancy.

Often the issue is raised of responding to the unwanted pregnancy by psychiatric treatment. The assessment of the usefulness and type of therapy should be a routine part of psychiatric evaluation. However, the recommenda-tion for therapy is in a large part independent of the decision about the abortion. It should be decided on its own merits by the usual criteria. One rather obvious factor is that time is important. That is, to delay abortion to see if therapy would be effective runs the risk of complicating both the psy-chological and physical problems of the abortion. Psychiatric treatment could be recommended either if abortion is recommended or thought advisable. Abortion should not be conditional on therapy in the future any more than it should be limited to women who have had therapy prior to requesting abortion. The former is coercive and the latter is discriminatory.

CONCLUSION

Nearly all authors not bound by religious or personal philosophy to an extreme position about therapeutic abortion have emphasized the need to assess each case on its own merits. The psychiatrist most interested in his patient's welfare will scrutinize himself thoroughly to avoid allowing his per-sonal value-systems to override the needs of the pregnant woman being considered for interruption.

The data that is available to assist in arriving at a decision about the interruption of pregnancy have been discussed in some detail in the preceding sections of the paper. Some concepts of Kummer[18] will be useful in this summary.

Therapeutic abortion should be considered when the woman displays a deep-seated conviction, arrived at on her own and not through pressure of spouse, family, friends, or physician, that the pregnancy is unwanted and intolerable, and she wishes to interrupt it; when the possibility exists that the woman would injure or kill herself; when the possibility exists of the woman injuring or killing others, particularly the newborn; when the problems related to management of the continuing pregnancy (hospitalization, restraint, care of the newborn) are so overwhelming, complicated and noxious in their own right that they make interruption a more therapeutic and practical choice; when continuation would result in extreme anguish as seen in a situation in which there is high risk of serious pathology in the child due to hereditary or congenital defect; when the psychiatric illness that might result would be of great length, difficult to treat and difficult to reverse; and when the pregnancy has been forced upon the woman through rape, or the woman's lack of awareness as in pregnancy of the very young or in mentally defectives.

SUMMARY

Psychological indications for therapeutic abortion are primarily related to the issue of the unwanted pregnancy. Of 249 Swedish women turned down for therapeutic abortion, 75 per cent had serious psychological problems related to the unwanted pregnancy during the eleven year follow-up period. A study of 125 children born to Swedish women turned down for therapeutic abortion and compared to matched controls, revealed a higher incidence of psychological and social problems in the study group. Despite conflicting claims, the best data available indicate a sizable number of women made suicide attempts while pregnant (7 per cent in a series of 497 women in Australia) and in about half of these the attempt was related in a significant way to the pregnancy.

Psychiatric diagnosis as such is not usually a major issue in determining indications or outome for therapeutic abortion. Over 200 American women studied by four different groups of investigators, and nearly 500 Swedish women studied by Ekblad, clearly demonstrate that women with a wide variety of psychiatric diagnoses experience therapeutic interruption of pregnancy as a positive event and very little new psychiatric pathology can be related to a therapeutic abortion. Other specific situations carrying sufficient morbid risk to justify termination of pregnancy especially where the mother desires it include incest, adolescent pregnancy, the possibility of serious hereditary defects in the child, and a history of postpartum psychosis.

REFERENCES

1. Adams, M. S., and Neel, J. V.: Children of incest. Pediatrics 40:55-62, 1967.

2. Anderson, E. W.: Psychiatric indications for termination of pregnancy. J. Psychosom. Res. 10:123-134, 1966.

3. Anthony, E. J.: A group of murderous mothers. Acta Psychother. 7: 1–6, 1959.

4. Aren, P.: Account in Year Book of Obstetrics and Gynecology. Chicago, Year Book Medical Publishers, 1958–1959, p. 64.

5. ——, and Amark, C.: The prognosis in which legal abortion has been granted but not carried out. Acta. Psychiat. et Neurol. 36:203-278, 1961.

6. Brew, M. F., and Seidenberg, R.: Psychotic reactions associated with pregnancy and childbirth. J. Nerv. Ment. Dis. 3:408, 1950.

7. Carter, C. O.: Risk to offspring of incest. Lancet 1:436, 1967.

8. Clark, M., Forstner, I., Pond, D. A., and Tredgold, R. F.: Sequels of unwanted pregnancy: A follow up of patients referred for psychiatric opinion. Lancet 2:501-503, 1968.

9. Cushner, M. D.: Abortion and the law, Maryland. C. M. D. 36:9, 757-671, 1969.

10. Ekblad, N.: Induced abortion on psychiatric grounds. Acta Psychiat. Scand. 97:1-238, 1955.

11. Forssman, H., and Thuwe, I.: One hundred and twenty children born after application for therapeutic abortion refused. Acta Psychiat. Scand. 42:71-88, 1966.

12. Granacher, M., as reported in Höök, K.: Refused abortion. Acta. Psychiat. Scand. 39 suppl. 68, 16-17, 1963.

13. Höök, K.: Refused abortion. Acta. Psychiat. Scand. 39:1-156, 1963.

14. Hoover, J. E.: Uniform Crime Reports, 1966. Washington, D.C., U.S. Gov. Printing Office, 1966.

15. Jansson, B.: Mental disorders after abortion. Acta. Psychiat. Scand. 41:87-110, 1965.

16. Jones, A. H.: Abortion and the law, North Carolina. C. M. D. 36:9, 751-752, 1969.

17. Kaufman, I., Peck, A., and Tagiuri, C.: The family constellation and overt incestuous relations between father and daughter. Amer. J. Orthopsychiat. 24:266-279, 1954.

18. Kummer, J. M.: Psychiatric contraindications to pregnancy: with reference to therapeutic abortion and sterilization. Calif. Med. 79:31-35, 1953.

19. Levene, H. I., and Rigney, F.: Law, preventive psychiatry and therapeutic abortion. Read at Annual APA meeting, 1969.

20. Lindberg, B. J., as reported in Höök, K.: Refused abortion. Acta Psychiat. Scand. 39:14-16, 1963.

21. Malmfors, K.: The problem of women seeking abortion. In Calderone, M. (Ed.): Abortion in U.S. New York, Harper & Row, 1958, pp. 133-135.

22. Martin, M. D.: Puerperal mental illness: a follow up study of 75 cases. Brit. J. 2:773-777, 1958.

23. McCoy, D.: The emotional reaction of women to therapeutic abortion and sterilization. J. Obstet. Gynec. Brit. Comm. 75:1054-1057, 1968.

24. Mehlan, K. J.: In Year Book of Obstetrics and Gynecology. Chicago, Year Book Medical Publishers, 1956, pp. 57-58.

25. Niswander, K. R., and Patterson, R. J.: Psychological reaction to therapeutic abortion: Subject patient response. Obstet. Gynec. 29:5, 702-706, 1967.

26. Patt, S., Rappaport, R., and Barglow, P.: Follow up of therapeutic abortion. Arch. Gen. Psychiat. 20:408-414, 1969.

27. Peck, A., and Marcus, H.: Psychiatric sequelae of therapeutic interruption of pregnancy. J. Nerv. Ment. Dis. 143:417-425, 1966.

28. Protheroe, C.: Puerperal psychoses: long-term study 1927-1961. Brit. J. Psychiat. 115:9-30, 1969.

29. Pugh, T. F., Jerath, B. K., Schmidt, W. M., and Reed, R. B.: Rates of mental disease related to child bearing. New Eng. J. Med. 268: 1224-1228, 1963.

30. Resnick, P.: Child murder by parents: A psychiatric review of filicide. Amer. J. Psychiat. 126:3, 325-334, 1969.

31.—: Murder of the new born: A psychiatric review of neonaticide. Read at Annual APA Meeting, 1969.

32. Sim, M.: Psychiatric disorders of pregnancy. J. Psychosom. Res. 12:95-100, 1968.

33. Simon, N. M., Rothman, D., and Senturia, A. G.: Psychiatric illness following therapeutic abortion. Amer. J. Psychiat. 124:59-65, 1967.

34. Sloane, P., and Karpinski, E.: Effects of incest on the participants. Amer. J. Orthopsychiat. 12:666-673, 1942.

35. Spector, A. B.: Abortion and the Law, Maryland. C.M.D. 36:756-777, 1969.

36. Tietz, C., and Lehfeldt, H.: Legal abortion in Eastern Europe. JAMA 175: 1149-1154, 1961.

37. Vanden Bergh, R. L.: Abortion and psychosis. Psychiat. Spectator 3:5-6, 1966.

38. Vestergaard, E.: Father-daughter incest. Nord. Tid. for Kriminalvid. 48:159-188, 1960.

39. Waters, J. L.: Pregnancy in young adolescents: a syndrome of failures. So. Med. J. 62:655–158, 1969.

40. Whitlock, F. A., and Edwards, J. E.: Pregnancy and attempted suicide. Compr. Psychiat. 9:1–12, 1968.

Fetal "Indications" for Termination of Pregnancy

By HENRY L. NADLER, M.D.

I N THE VAST MAJORITY OF INSTANCES in which pregnancies have
been terminated on the basis of a known or suspected malformation of the
fetus, legal requirements have forced listing the indication for abortion as
"threat to the life of the mother" rather than to the fetus. This has been due
to the fact that fetal indications for interruption of pregnancy are poorly
defined. Because of the lack of accurate data and appropriate guidelines dealing with this problem, this manuscript will attempt only to review the known
causes of fetal malformations and to outline the newer techniques which
permit precise detection of the "high risk fetus."

Although congenital malformations and structural defects present at birth
have been recorded from time immemorial, their true incidence is unknown,
and most figures differ greatly because of lack of precision in defining terms
and different methods of ascertaining data. It is probably safe to say that
2-4 per cent of all live-born infants have one or more significant congenital
malformations detectable during the newborn period.[11] This figure is doubled
by the end of the first year of life with the discovery of malformations not
apparent at birth. The incidence of congenital malformations appears to
be increasing in recent years, a fact which may be explained by better methods
of detection, a decrease in the incidence of other pathological conditions of
childhood, and finally increased survival of affected children.

Our knowledge of the specific etiology of the majority of congenital
malformations is sadly lacking. A general scheme of classification of causes
might include genetic factors, chromosomal factors, viral infections, environmental, and miscellaneous or unidentified causes. Estimates have suggested
that genetic factors might be responsible for approximately 20 per cent of all
malformations, chromosomal aberrations for 10-15 per cent, and viral infections
for 10 per cent, leaving somewhat more than 50 per cent unidentified and
presumably due to other causes.[27]

Over two thousand conditions have been described in which genetic factors
presumably play a role.[13] The genetic basis may be either simple or complex.
Many genetic disorders are inherited directly through either one or both of
the parents. The common modes of inheritance include autosomal dominant,
autosomal recessive, X-linked recessive and X-linked dominant. In dominant
conditions one parent may be affected and carry the particular mutant gene,
transmitting it to one-half of his children; or, the mutant gene may have
arisen spontaneously as a new mutation. Disorders inherited in this manner
include achondroplasia, mandibulo facial dysostosis, Marfan's syndrome and
many others. Many of the common skeletal malformation syndromes are
inherited in this fashion.

Congenital malformations may be inherited as recessive genes in which both
parents are normal but each carries one mutant gene and one normal gene

for a particular trait. In these conditions the parents' risk of having a child with the particular malformation is one in four. Conditions inherited in this fashion include types of chondrodystrophies, Morquio's syndrome, polycystic kidneys—juvenile form and many biochemical disorders leading to mental retardation or death in early infancy.

Unfortunately, complex genetic factors are responsible for many congenital malformations, and the risks in future pregnancies do not follow classic genetic ratios. Cleft lip and palate, anencephaly, club foot, congenital dislocation of the hip, hydrocephalus, and certain types of congenital heart disease are inherited in this fashion.

The relationship of chromosomal aberrations to congenital malformations has been recognized for only 10 years. The first congenital malformation syndrome in which a chromosome aberration was shown to be the cause was Down's syndrome (mongolism), a disorder in which characteristic facial features are associated with mental deficiency.[8] Down's syndrome occurs with a frequency of 1/600 live births. The frequency of this disorder has been shown to be directly related to the age of the mother. The likelihood of a woman at age 25 years of having a child with Down's syndrome is approximately 1/2500, at age 35 1/250, age 40 1/100 and age 45 1/50.[22] Similar maternal age effects are true for most other chromosomal aberrations. The vast majority of infants with Down's syndrome simply have an extra chromosome, i.e. 47, and most women having such a child are not at significantly increased risk of having a second. On occasion, this disorder is not a random event related to maternal age but is inherited from either one of the parents who carries a chromosome rearrangement. The risks in these cases is anywhere from 10-100 per cent. There are many other chromosome determined congenital malformation syndromes, many associated with mental retardation. A chromosomal aberration may be found in approximately 1 per cent of all live births.[3] In addition, about 25-40 per cent of spontaneous abortions occurring in the first three months of pregnancy are caused by a chromosomal aberration.[1]

Various drugs administered during pregnancy have been thought to be responsible for the appearance of congenital defects. The most widely studied and best documented example of a drug responsible for congenital malformation is thalidomide.[10] This drug, an efficient sedative, has been incriminated in producing specific congenital deformities including reduction deformities of the limbs, hypoplasia of the ear and congenital heart defects. This agent, taken at most times during pregnancy, apparently has no harmful effects to the fetus; however, when taken at a specific time early in pregnancy the risk to the fetus approaches 100 per cent.[9] Other drugs incriminated in producing deformities are listed in Table 1. This subject has recently been reviewed by McKay and Lucey,[12] and Smithells.[25]

Viral infections have been held responsible for the production of congenital malformation.[24] The relationship of one specific virus, rubella or German measles, to congenital malformations has been precisely defined during the past 30 years.[2,7] Children born to mothers who have had German measles during early pregnancy may have multiple malformations including cataracts,

Table 1.—Medications Presumably Capable of Causing Congenital Malformations

Maternal Medication*	Fetal Defect
Thalidomide	Phocomelia, hearing loss and fetal death
Oral progestins, androgens, and estrogens	Masculinization and advanced bone age
Antimetabolites, including aminopterin, amethopterin, chlorambucil	Anomalies and abortions
Potassium iodide, propylthiouracil, mehimazole	Goiter
Bishydroxycoumarin	Fetal death and hemorrhage
Sulfonylurea derivatives	Anomalies (?)
Chloroquine	Retinal damage or death (?)
Antihistamines	Anomalies (?)

*Many other agents have effects upon the fetus but do not result in malformation.

heart disease, deafness, microcephaly, mental deficiency, bone and liver disease. The specific time in pregnancy in which the infection occurs determines the degree and extent of the malformations. Infection in the first two months of pregnancy is more likely to result in deformities to the fetus than infection in the third and fourth months. Infection in the third and fourth and even fifth months still carries specific and well defined risks to the fetus. This viral infection was responsible for the birth of approximately 8000 infants with malformations after the 1964 epidemic of German measles. Other infectious agents suspected or proven to cause congenital malformations are listed in Table 2.[24]

Fetal irradiation has been recognized to produce congenital deformities for many years. Almost all of these cases followed the use of large doses of X-ray or radiation to treat malignancies of pregnant women.[15] Therapeutic pelvic irradiation during pregnancy has essentially ceased and is of limited concern. More recently, evidence has been presented suggesting that certain congenital deformities are increased in the infants of mothers exposed to radiation from atomic fallout.[23,28] This clearly may represent a real risk in future generations. While the dangers of large doses of radiation to the embryo are recognized,

Table 2.—Infections Causing Malformations in the Fetus or Newborn

Maternal Infection	Effects on Fetus or Newborn
Rubella	Malformations, bleeding, hepatitis, encephalitis, etc.
Cytomegalovirus	Microcephaly, chorioretinitis, deafness and mental retardations
Mumps	Fetal death, endocardial fibroelastosis (?) and malformations
Rubeola	Increased abortion and stillbirths
Varicella	Increased abortion and stillbirths
Vaccinia	Increased abortion and stillbirths
Influenza	Malformations(?)
Syphilis	Congenital syphilis
Listeriosis	Abortions and stillbirths, habitual abortions(?)
Toxoplasmosis	Microcephaly, chorioretinitis, jaundice, etc.

Modified from Sever.[12]

the relationship of low doses of radiation to congenital malformations is unknown. There is no evidence to suggest that diagnostic X ray to the nonpregnant woman carries any significant risk to the fetus.

The relationship of the environment to congenital malformations and genetic disorders is one in which increasing attention has recently been focused. The difficulty in this type of study is primarily that of identification of the offending agent. For example, if a drug were to be responsible for a one-tenth of 1 per cent increase in the incidence of a particular common congenital deformity, it would be difficult, if not impossible, to detect this relationship. Clearly, methods of testing the mutagenic capabilities of new drugs, as well as other environmental agents, must be developed.

During recent years, the development of specialized surgical, orthopedic, medical and physical rehabilitative techniques have led to significant modification of the tragic consequences of many congenital malformations. The toll in terms of financial cost to parents and society, as well as the problems for the affected patient, are great. Many birth defects have, at present, no successful therapy available to modify the natural history of the disease. Clearly, the challenge of the future lies in the development of techniques to prevent birth defects.

Prevention can be dealt with in many ways, depending upon the specific cause. Rubella should disappear as a major cause of congenital malformations with the distribution of the recently developed vaccines.[14] Vaccines should be developed to prevent the sequelae of other viruses and infectious agents which might produce deformities of unborn babies.

Genetic counseling may be effective when congenital malformation syndromes are recognized and called to the attention of the family. Laboratory tests including chromosome analysis, biochemical tests and tissue culture techniques have been developed which permit precise identification of the parents at increased risk of having a child with a genetic defect and genetic counseling could theoretically be effective.

Recently, it has become possible to detect a number of significant genetic disorders and birth defects in utero. The ability to detect an affected fetus in utero provides a new precision to genetic counseling. It enables couples who would normally not hazard the risks of having a defective child to have normal children. Disorders which have been detected early in pregnancy and in which abortion might be considered include chromosomal aberrations,[16,17,26] X-linked uric aciduria,[4] mucopolysaccharidosis,[6,16] cystic fibrosis,[18] deficiency of lysosomal acid phosphatase,[19] Pompe's disease,[20] and galactosemia.[16] Many other disorders have been shown to have an abnormal phenotype in tissue culture and therefore theoretically could be detected in utero.[17] In fact, families with a number of these disorders have had pregnacies successfully managed and normal children delivered. The technique of transabdominal amniocentesis has been performed between the twelfth and twentieth week in over 350[4] cases as part of the management of genetic "high risk" pregnancies.[21] In our experience neither fetal or maternal morbidity or mortality has been observed.

The following cases are examples of pregnancies which have been interrupted because of congenital malformations of the fetus:

Case 1. A 26-year-old carrier of a chromosomal rearrangement, D/G translocation, had a transabdominal amniocentesis performed at 14 weeks of pregnancy. Chromosome analysis of cultivated amniotic fluid cells revealed a karyotype consistent with Down's syndrome-translocation type. The pregnancy was terminated at 18 weeks of gestation.

Case 2. A 43-year-old female had had an amniocentesis performed at 15 weeks because of maternal age. Chromosome analysis of cultivated amniotic fluid cells demonstrated 47 chromosomes, including an extra "G" chromosome, consistent with trisomic Down's syndrome. The pregnancy was terminated at 19 weeks of gestation.

Case 3. A 27-year-old female who was a D/G translocation carrier was referred by her obstetrician four and a half years ago. On the basis of a risk of 10-30 per cent of having another child with Down's syndrome the parents requested termination of a pregnancy. The pregnancy was terminated at eight weeks of pregnancy.

Case 4. A 32-year-old mother, with three normal children, had a documented rubella infection at five weeks of pregnancy. Based upon the "high" risk of the fetus being affected, the parents elected to have the pregnancy terminated.

Case 5. A 27-year-old mother developed acute toxoplasmosis at 16 days of pregnancy. Serological confirmation was obtained and the family elected to have the pregnancy terminated.

Case 6. This family was referred at six weeks of pregnancy because of a history of having two children with congenital deafness. The parents were not prepared to chance another child with deafness and wished the pregnancy terminated.

Case 7. This mother had previously delivered two boys with Duchenne type muscular dystrophy (X-linked recessive) and wished to have a normal child. Amniocentesis was performed at 15 weeks of pregnancy and the sex of fetus determined to be a male. On the basis of a 50 per cent chance of being affected, the parents requested termination of the pregnancy.

The preceding cases demonstrate the problems encountered when one discusses fetal "indications" for abortion. In the first two cases, intrauterine diagnosis established that the fetus in fact had Down's syndrome. These cases would be easily handled by most physicians and parents. The problem of detecting a disorder in which the handicaps are less severe might cause more difficulty. What is the "minimum" handicap which would be an acceptable indication for both parents and physicians to consider interruption of pregnancy?

In Cases 3, 4, and 7, although intrauterine detection of the disorder was not possible, the risks were significant enough for the family to elect termination of pregnancy.

In Case 5, a more difficult problem was encountered. Toxoplasmosis has been known to be related to congenital malformations for many years, however, the precise risk to the baby at specific times in gestation is not known with the same certainty as rubella. Prospective studies by Desmonts[5] and Sever[24] have suggested that the risk might be in the order of 20 per cent. Desmonts points out that no case of congenital toxoplasmosis was found when maternal infection preceded pregnancy. Was the patient in Case 5 at increased risk or not? After consultations with a number of physicians the family elected to terminate the pregnancy.

When therapeutic abortion is considered for potential fetal malformation, the questions which arise are difficult, if not impossible, to answer. What is a significant "risk" or a significant "malformation"? Many abortions could be prevented simply by effective contraception. The family who wants more children but does not wish to risk another defective child can be easily managed if intrauterine diagnosis is possible. When intrauterine diagnosis is not possible, then contraception or acceptance of the risk are the possible choices.

The difficult problems arise in either cases of exposure to "infectious agents or teratogens" which might be capable of producing congenital malformations or when the disorder is not associated with significant mental retardation, morbidity or mortality. The ultimate decision as to how these patients can be counseled and treated probably depends upon clear definition of abortion laws. If abortion becomes the right of any woman, the problem is readily solved. However, if abortions laws attempt to define which malformations of the fetus are to be considered indications for abortions, a tremendous grey zone will remain in which patients will be handled as they have been during the past decades.

Summary

The premise of this discussion is that fetal "indications" for abortion do exist. However, the precise definition of these indications is difficult, if not impossible. When definitive detection of disorders in which "significant" mental retardation, morbidity or mortality can be accomplished in utero, arguments against abortion can only be presented on "moral" grounds. In cases where specific risk figures are available, few arguments are encountered. The greatest difficulty is with disorders in which there are "minimal" risks for malformations or in which the defects are compatible with normal life span but carry different degrees of morbidity. This last group is impossible to define precisely, and probably only laws which permit abortion at the request of the mother can provide useful guidelines.

REFERENCES

1. Carr, D. H.: Chromosome anomalies as a cause of spontaneous abortion. Amer. J. Obstet. Gynec. 97:283–293, 1967.

2. Cooper, L. Z., and Krugman, S.: Diagnosis and management: congenital rubella. Pediatrics 37:335–338, 1966.

3. Court Brown, W. M.: Population Cytogenetics. Amsterdam, North Holland Publishing, 1967.

4. DeMars, R., Sarto, G., Felix, J. S., and Benke, P.: Lesch-Nyhan mutation: prenatal detection with amniotic fluid cells. Science 164:1303–1305, 1969.

5. Desmonts, G., Couvreur, J., and Ben-Rachid, M. S.: Le toxoplasme, la mere et l'enfant. Arch. Franc Pediat. 22:1183–1200, 1965.

6. Frantantoni, J. C., Neufeld, E. F., Uhlendorf, B. W., and Jacobson, C. B.: Intra-uterine diagnosis of the Hurler's and Hunter's syndromes. New Eng. J. Med. 280: 686–688, 1969.

7. Gregg, H. M.: Congenital cataract following German measles in mother. Trans. Ophthal. Soc. Aus. 3:35–46, 1941.

8. Lejeune, J., Gautier, M., and Turpin, R.: Etude des chromosomes somatiques de neuf enfants mongoliens. C. R. Acad. Sci. 248:1721, 1959.

9. Lenz, W. (cited by Taussig, H. B.): A study of the German outbreak of phocomelia. The thalidomide syndrome. JAMA 180:1106–1114, 1962.

10. Lenz, W.: Chemicals and malformations in man. Second Inter. Conference on Congenital Malformations. New York, The International Medical Congress, 1964, pp. 263–276.

11. McIntosh, R., Marritt, K. K., Richards, M. R., Samuels, M. H., and Bellows, M. T.: Incidence of congenital malformations: study of 5964 pregnancies. Pediatrics 15:505–521, 1954.

12. McKay, R. J., Jr., and Lucey, J. F.: Neonatology. New Eng. J. Med. 270:1231–1236, 1964.

13. McKusick, V. A.: Mendelian Inheritance in Man (ed.2). Baltimore, Johns Hopkins Press, 1968.

14. Meyer, H. M., Parkman, P. D., and Panos, T. C.: Attenuated rubella virus: II. production of experimental live-virus vaccine and clinical trial. New Eng. J. Med. 275:575–580, 1966.

15. Murphy, D. P.: Outcome of 625 pregnancies in women subjected to pelvic radium or roentgen irradiation. Amer. J. Obstet. Gynec. 18:179–187, 1929.

16. Nadler, H. L.: Antenatal detection of hereditary disorders. Pediatrics 42:912–918, 1968.

17. —: Medical progress. Prenatal detection of genetic defects. J. Pediat. 72:132–143, 1969.

18. —, Swae, M., Wodnicki, J., and O'Flynn, M. E.: Cultivated amniotic fluid cells and fibroblasts derived from families with cystic fibrosis. Lancet 2:84–85, 1969.

19. —, and Egan, T. J.: Lysosomal acid phosphatase deficiency: a new familial metabolic disorder. New Eng. J. Med. 282: 302–307, 1970.

20. —, and Messina, A. M.: in utero detection of Type II glycogenosis (Pompe's Disease). Lancet 2:1277–1278, 1969.

21. —, and Gerbie, A. B.: The Role of Amniocentesis in the intra-uterine detection of Genetic Disorders. New Eng. J. Med. 282:596–599, 1970.

22. Penrose, L. S., and Smith, G. F.: Down's Anomaly. Boston, Little, Brown, 1966, p. 157.

23. Plummer, G.: Anomalies occurring in children exposed in utero to atomic bomb in Hiroshima. Pediatrics 10:687–692, 1952.

24. Sever, J. L.: Perinatal infections affecting the developing fetus and newborn. In Eichenwald, H. F. (Ed.): The Prevention of Mental Retardation Through Control of Infectious Diseases. Bethesda, United States Public Service, National Institute of Child Health and Development.

25. Smithells, R. W.: Drugs and human malformations. In Woollam, D. H. M. (Ed.): Advances in Teratology, Vol. I (ed.1). London, Logos Press, 1966.

26. Valenti, C., Schutta, E. J., and Kehaty, T.: Prenatal diagnosis of Down's syndrome. Lancet 2:220, 1968.

27. Warkany, J., and Kalter, H.: Medical progress. Congenital malformations. New Eng. J. Med. 265:993–1001, 1046-1052, 1961.

28. Yamazaki, J. N., Wright, S. W., and Wright, P. M.: Outcome of pregnancy in women exposed to atomic bomb in Nagasaki. Amer. J. Dis. Child. 87:448–463, 1954.

Abortion Attitudes of Poverty-Level Blacks

By Clark E. Vincent, Ph.D., C. Allen Haney, Ph.D., and Carl M. Cochrane, Ph.D.

T HE PURPOSE OF THIS PAPER is the modest one of presenting information about the attitudes of poverty-level blacks concerning abortion. The descriptive rather than analytic manner in which the data and discussion are presented is due to the fact that only preliminary analyses of the data have been completed at this time. The paucity of existing information about poverty-level blacks' attitudes concerning abortion, and the opportunity of comparing our findings on blacks with the National Opinion Research Center data for whites, were believed to justify this preliminary and descriptive report of information derived from a much larger study of knowledge, attitudes, and practices of poverty-level blacks concerning family planning.

DATA COLLECTION PROCEDURES

Population and Sample

Six contiguous census tracts containing the highest proportion of poverty-level black residents in a Standard Metropolitan Statistical Area in North Carolina were selected as the base population from which the study was derived. These six tracts contained approximately 5500 poverty-level black females of child-bearing age. The sample within these six census tracts consisted of every fifth consecutively numbered dwelling unit, except that for every fifth consecutively numbered block all dwelling units were included on a saturation basis. If a dwelling unit contained more than one household (4%), and if more than one eligible female lived in the same household (5%), all eligible females in that household were interviewed. Eligibility as a respondent necessitated being a black female between the ages of 15-39, having had at least one pregnancy, and being at the poverty-level (using our modification of Orshansky's Index[2]) (see appendix).

This sampling procedure resulted in usable interviews with 776 poverty-level black females who were well within our modification of Orshansky's definition of poverty. During the pretesting of the interview schedule, the questions used to establish the poverty-level status of the respondent were asked at the beginning of the interview. However, because the respondents interpreted this early focus on income questions as evidence that the study was welfare sponsored and possibly related to "welfare investigations," the income items were placed at the end of the interview. As a result of this change, our final study group included an additional 215 females with a mean annual household income of $7500, and a group of 88 females whose annual household income placed them midway between the poverty-level group of

---

Supported in part by grants from the Ford Foundation and from The Welfare and Social Security Administrations, United States Department of Health, Education, and Welfare (CRD-283 and H-273).

Table 1.—Selected Characteristics of a Poverty-Level Group and Lower-Middle
Income Group of Black Females

Characteristics	PL Group (N=776)	LMI Group (N=215)
Median household income	$2522	$7775
Per cent with income under $3000	64%	0%
Per cent with ADC as major source of income	44%	4%
Per cent with 12 years of education	30%	59%
Median years of school completed	10.3 yrs.	11.7 yrs.
Per cent not working at present	80%	41%
Mean age of respondent	26.6	24.8
Mean number of persons in household	6.1	5.2
Per cent of households with spouse present	25%	57%
Per cent of households with no male adult	62%	15%
Mean number of children in household	4.3	2.6

776 and the "lower middle income" group of 215. The group of 88 females are excluded from the present report. A summary of selected characteristics for the poverty level (PL) group of 776 and the lower middle income (LMI) group of 215 is shown in Table 1. A more detailed report of sampling and interviewing procedures is contained elsewhere.[9]

Interviewing Procedures

In selecting persons to interview the respondents for two-and-a-half to three hours, high priority was given those able to converse comfortably in the general vernacular and specific sex terminology of poverty-level blacks. The interviewers worked in teams of two, usually one black and one white female, which made it possible for one interviewer to conduct the interview while the other one contained or minimized interruptions from children, or simply waited outside to provide implicit protection in some of the rougher neighborhoods. The team approach also facilitated simultaneous but independent interviews of two eligible females in the same household. One black husband-wife team and one black brother-sister team were used to obtain interview data from approximately 500 of the females' husbands and/or current sexual partners.

GENERAL FINDINGS

The initial item on abortion attitudes was prefaced by the interviewer's statement "Some pregnant women get abortions." The respondent was then asked "How do you feel about this?" and was asked to give the reasons "why" she felt as she did. Later the respondent was also asked to report on the attitudes about abortion held by her mother, her maternal grandmother, and her husband or current sexual partner.

The proportion of respondents opposed to abortions was much higher than expected (Table 2); 86 per cent of the 500 males, 79 per cent of the PL females and 70 per cent of the LMI group were not in favor of abortions under any circumstances. Only 14 of the 776 PL subjects, one of the 215 LMI

Table 2.—Distribution of Attitudes About Abortion for Two Socioeconomic
Groups of Black Females, and One Group of Black Males

| Attitudes and Rationale | Females[*] | | Males[*] |
	PL Grow (N=776)	LMI Group (N=215)	(N=500)
Opposed to Abortion (%)			
Religious reasons only ("not right")	42	35	57
Health reasons only ("dangerous")	21	17	12
Religious and health reasons	16	18	17
Favorable to Abortion (%)			
If for health reasons (of mother)	17	27	1
Unqualified	2	00	13
Other (No opinion or contradictory response)	2	3	–
	100%	100%	100%

[*]See Table 1 for description of two groups of females. The males were predominantely the husbands or current sexual partners of the PL group of females. See Table 3 for educational distribution.

subjects, and 7 of the 500 males expressed unqualified approval of abortion. The one consistently given reason for even qualified approval of abortion was "mother's health," which most frequently was on a life or death basis.

Education

The anticipated positive relation between educational level and opinions on abortion (Table 3) was found for both groups of females, as well as for the males. As was also expected, increased education in all three groups was inversely related to religious reasons ("not right") for being opposed to abortions.

For the females, the directional trend of the relation between having less education and giving "dangerous to mother's health" as a reason for negative attitudes toward abortion may reflect the predominance of "do-it-yourself" methods of abortion among the poor and uneducated, methods that are dangerous at best and range from overdoses of harsh laxatives to inserting a garden hose into the vagina and against the opening of the cervix.[*] As Lee has documented, the search for an abortionist can be highly complex and involved even for college-educated females with sufficient money.[1]

Race and Education

Some education and race comparisons are possible between our findings and those of Rossi[5,6] that were obtained from a representative sample of 1484

---

[*]The wide variety and the frequent use of "home remedies" and the folk methods for abortion that were discovered indirectly in the present study are documented in a series of as yet unpublished AFDC studies conducted at the Institute for Social Research of Florida State University (Welfare Administration Grant No. 155).

Table 3.–Distribution of Opinions on Abortion for Two Socioeconomic Groups of Black Females and One Group of Black Males by Education

| | Females | | | | | | | | Males (N=500) | | | |
| | PL Group (N=757)* | | | | LMI Group (N=206)* | | | | | | | |
Attitudes and Rationale	Eighth Grade or Less (N=136)	Some High School (N=391)	Completed High School (N=185)	Some College or More (N=45)	Eighth Grade or Less (N=10)	Some High School (N=73)	Completed High School (N=80)	Some College or More (N=43)	Eighth Grade or Less (N=99)	Some High School (N=200)	Completed High School (N=147)	Some College or More (N=54)
Opposed to Abortion (%)												
Religious Reasons Only	49	45	40	22	40	41	39	25	70	58	57	46
Health Reasons Only	23	22	19	20	30	16	15	19	8	11	16	7
Religious and Health Reasons	16	15	17	25	20	22	15	16	18	19	13	19
Favorable (%) (Qualified and Unqualified)†	12	18	24	33	10	21	31	40	5	13	14	28
	100%	100%	100%	100%	100%	100%	100%	100%	101%	101%	100%	100%

*Numbers are slightly smaller than reported in Table 2, due to lack of education data for some respondents.
†"Qualified" and "unqualified" combined, since less than 2 per cent in the latter category.

adult Americans via a National Opinion Research Center survey in December, 1965. In the Rossi study the respondents were asked:

"Please tell me whether or not you think it should be possible for a pregnant woman to obtain a legal abortion. . . ." in each of six specified circumstances: "mother's health," "rape," "defects in fetus," "poor," "unmarried," "married but wants no more children."

Our item did not specify the circumstances but probed for the reasons why the respondent felt either opposed or favorable to the fact that "some women get abortions." Since the circumstance of "mother's health" was associated with the highest percentage of Rossi's respondents favoring abortion and was the consistent reason given by those of our respondents favoring abortion, the comparisons shown in Table 4 seem appropriate. These comparisons understate the actual differences in the findings of the two studies, because the percentages for the North Carolina study of blacks represent the totals of all respondents favoring abortions under any circumstances while the percentages for Rossi's representative study of whites[7] represent only those favoring abortions for reasons of the mother's health.

In each of the four educational groupings compared in Table 4, the proportion of white males in the NORC study favoring abortion was at least 50 percentage points higher than for the black males in our study; the proportion of white females in the NORC study favoring abortion was never less than 35 percentage points higher than for the black females in our PL and LMI groups.

Additional comparisons may be made between our findings and those of Peyton, et al.[3] who used a mail-questionnaire to study 2070 gynecological, private-practice patients "primarily Caucasian, middle class, permanent residents of west central Indiana." For their total respondents 80 per cent would justify abortion if the mother's life were endangered; 74 per cent and 76 per cent respectively would justify abortion if the mother's physical or mental health were seriously impaired.

Table 4.—Respondents in Two Studies Who Believe Mother's Health
Acceptable Reason for Abortion

Study	Males				Females			
	8th Grade or Less	Some High School	Completed High School	Some College or More	8th Grade or Less	Some High School	Completed High School	Some College or More
NORC (Rossi) (%)*	57	76	79	81	66	64	75	75
N=	(241)	(140)	(165)	(166)	(160)	(219)	(200)	(180)
North Carolina PL Group	5	13	14	28	12	18	24	33
N=	(99)	(200)	(147)	(54)	(136)	(391)	(185)	(45)
LMI Group	—	—	—	—	10	21	31	40
N=	(−)	(−)	(−)	(−)	(10)	(73)	(80)	(43)

*From A. S. Rossi: Public views on abortions, in Guttmacher, A. F., (Ed.) The Case for Legalized Abortion Now. Berkeley, Diablo Press, 1967, p. 38, Table 2.

Table 5.—Distribution of Attitudes about Abortion for Two Socioeconomic Groups of Black Females

Attitudes and Rationale	Church Membership				Frequency of Church Attendance					
	PL Group		LMI Group		PL Group			LMI Group		
	No (N=96)	Yes (N=667)	No (N=9)	Yes (N=198)	Low* (N=119)	Medium† (N=242)	High‡ (N=380)	Low* (N=15)	Medium† (N=70)	High‡ (N=115)
Opposed to Abortion (%)										
Religious Reasons Only	46	42	33	36	52	42	41	27	24	45
Health Reasons Only	25	21	11	17	17	23	22	13	19	15
Religions and Health Reasons	16	17	33	18	18	15	18	27	19	16
Favorable (%) (Qualified and Unqualified)†	14	20	22	29	13	20	19	33	38	23
	101%	100%	99%	100%	100%	100%	100%	100%	100%	99%

*Never or once or twice a year
†Once or twice a month
‡Three or more times a month

Church Membership and Attendance

The church affiliations of our poverty-level sample were Baptist (59%), Holiness (15%), Methodist (10%), "none" (12%), and "other" (4%). We had anticipated that church membership and greater frequency of church attendance would be associated with religious rationale for those negative attitudes, but the findings generally were in the opposite direction. Of 667 PL females with church membership, 80 per cent were opposed to abortion and 42 per cent gave religious reasons for such opposition; of 96 PL females not belonging to any church 86 per cent were opposed to abortion and 46 per cent gave religious reasons for their attitude. For the PL females with "high frequency" (three or more per month) of church attendance, 81 per cent were opposed to abortion, and 41 per cent gave religious reasons. For the PL females with "low frequency" (never or several times a year) of church attendance, 87 per cent were opposed to abortion; 52 per cent gave religious reasons (Table 5).

Although not significant, the directional trend of the findings for the PL females was contrary to what we expected, and to Rossi's findngs. Rossi found that high church attendance (several times a month or more) was strongly associated with conservative views on abortion, and that the variable of church attendance accounted for a good deal of the difference between Catholics and Protestants and between males and females on views toward abortion.[8]

For the LMI group the number not belonging to a church (9) is too small for comparative purposes, but the trend of the relation between frequency of church attendance and attitudes about abortion is in the same direction as that reported by Rossi. For LMI females with high frequency of church attendance, 77 per cent were opposed to abortion and 45 per cent gave religious

Table 6.—Church Membership and Frequency of Church Attendance for Two Socioeconomic Groups of Black Females

		PL Group Educational Attainment			LMI Group Educational Attainment	
		8 years or less	9–11 Years	12 years or more	Less Than 12th Grade§	12th Grade or more§
Church Membership		(N=135)	(N=390)	(N=236)	(N=83)	(N=125)
No		21	12	9	7	2
Yes		79	88	91	93	98
	Total	100%	100%	100%	100%	100%
Church Attendance		(N=135)	(N=375)	(N=231)	(N=80)	(N=120)
Low*		23	18	9	9	6
Medium†		31	33	33	33	37
High‡		46	49	58	58	57
	Total	100%	100%	100%	100%	100%

*Never, or once or twice a year
†Once or twice a month
‡Three or more times a month
§Educational categories were combined because of the small numbers who were not church members,[9] and had low church attendance.[15]

reasons. The comparative percentages for the LMI females with low frequency of church attendance were 67 per cent and 27 per cent.

Education was clearly and consistently associated with both church membership and frequency of church attendance for the PL group, but less so for the LMI group (Table 6). The interrelation of education, church membership and attendance, and attitudes about abortion is a complex one that will be explored in subsequent analyses of the data.

Summary

The preliminary examination of frequency distributions of the attitudes about abortion expressed by a sample of 776 poverty level (PL) and 215 lower middle income (LMI) black females, ages 15 to 39, revealed no association of their attitudes with age, parity, marital status, and "miscarriages" (spontaneous and induced).

Much higher proportions (80-87 per cent) of these two groups of black females, as well as of 500 of their husbands and/or current sexual partners, were found to be opposed to abortion than has been found for predominantly white respondents (20-35 per cent).

The positive and consistent association between education and favorable attitudes about abortion, which we found for both groups of black females and for the black males, is consistent with similar findings by others for whites.

The trend of our findings that favorable attitudes of blacks about abortion were positively related to church membership and to frequency of church attendance was in the opposite direction from previous findings for whites. Rossi, for example, found that for whites frequent church attendance was strongly associated with conservative views on abortion. However, our findings are consistent with those of Reiss[4] who found higher frequency of church attendance for blacks (but not for whites) to be associated with permissive premarital sexual attitudes.

The unexpected proportion of blacks in our study who expressed highly conservative views on abortion is contrary to the general consensus of the existing literature that Blacks' sexual behavior and attitudes are more permissive than those of whites. Whether these more conservative views are limited to abortion, or are also present in regards to other sexually-related behavior for our study groups will be explored in subsequent analyses of the data. Further exploration of the initial finding of a directional trend between increased frequency of church attendance and more liberal attitudes about abortion may reveal this seemingly contrary trend to be related to the educational level of frequent church attenders. The preliminary stage of our data analysis at this time, however, has precluded other than descriptive reporting of the results of initial data runs and frequency distributions on selected items.

Appendix

Poverty levels were determined by the relationship of income to family size. A set of income standards was calculated for each family size. This set of calculations assumed a minimum necessary income of $1900 for a single individual, $2700 for a couple, $3200 for a three person household, and approximately $600-$700 for each additional member of the household. Following this procedure, the poverty-level (PL) group of 776 females includes all respondents with a total family income of less than the foregoing standard with corresponding family size. The "lower-middle income" (LMI) group of 215 females consists of all respondents whose total family income was a minimum of $1500 above the foregoing standard for the PL group.

REFERENCES

1. Lee, N. H.: The Search for an Abortionist. Chicago, University of Chicago Press, 1969.

2. Orshansky, M.: Counting the poor: another look at the poverty profile. Social Security Bulletin 3–29, 1965.

3. Peyton, F. W., Starry, A. R., and Leidy, T. R.: Women's attitudes concerning abortion. Obstet. Gynec. 34:182–188, 1969.

4. Reiss, I. L.: The Social Context of Premarital Sexual Permissiveness. New York, Holt, Rinehart and Winston, 1967, pp. 49–51.

5. Rossi, A. S.: Public views on abortion. In Guttmacher, A. F. (Ed.): The Case for Legalized Abortion Now. Berkeley, Diablo Press, 1967, pp. 26–53.

6.—: Abortion laws and their victims. Transaction 3:7–12, 1966.

7. —: Personal communication.

8. —: Public views on abortion. In Guttmacher, A. F. (Ed.): The Case for Legalized Abortion Now. Berkeley, Diablo Press, 1967, p. 44.

9. Vincent, C. E., Haney, C. A., and Cochrane, C. M.: Familial and generational patterns of illegitimacy. Journal of Marriage and the Family. 31:659–667, 1969.

Socioeconomic Aspects of Abortion

By David Goldberg, M.A., M.R.C.P., D.P.M

IN RECENT YEARS, while the number of medical indications for abortion has been shrinking[25] and the traditional psychiatric indications called to question,[6,60,61] progressively more abortions have been performed for social and socioeconomic indications.[56,64] In countries where abortions are permitted only for medical indications it is common for social indications to masquerade as psychiatric illnesses,[46,47] and it is of interest that in a previous book written mainly by psychiatrists about abortion,[58] socioeconomic conditions are only discussed by Guttmacher,[25] who is himself an obstetrician. He writes:

> In our country (U.S.A.) in the year 1953, socio-economic conditions *per se* never warrant therapeutic abortion. It is only human that they may weigh heavily in the scale when other factors bring about consideration of abortion. For example, one is more prone to abort the cardiac patient who is unwed, on relief and already mother of several children, than the woman with the same degree of cardiac pathology who is married, childless and well-to-do. Still, with the established code of ethics for the medical profession, no socio-economic situation, no matter how crying, alone justifies evacuation of an early pregnancy.

Attitudes have changed since 1953, and some psychiatrists have argued that social factors are relevant since they influence the mental state:

> A woman with an alcoholic husband, seven children, no friends, and arrears of rent has social problems which cannot fail to influence the mental state, and hence the justification for therapeutic abortion. If there is one lesson to be learned from fifty years research it is that social and mental health are inseparable . . .[19]

Others have been more outspoken, and argued for a direct assessment of social factors without necessarily referring to the mental state. Sloane[61] writes: "the problem of advising abortion for psychiatric grounds is far more often the question of judging the effect of the addition of another child to a household or mother, or both, under stress than predicting the likelihood of madness or suicide."

In countries such as Norway,[41] Finland,[33,54] Czechoslovakia,[40,66] Poland,[9] Hungary,[49] and Japan[44,62] abortions are allowed for such purely social reasons as housing problems and economic hardship. In nearly all of these surveys the majority of the abortions were carried out for social indications. Chroscielewski[9] reports that in Poland in 1964 there were 53 abortions for social indications for each one for a medical indication. In Hungary, where Mitenyi[49] reports that almost a third of abortions in his series are done for economic reasons, 15 per cent of the patients said that they wished to "better themselves and then have children" after the abortion. At Helsinki, Ingman[33] reports that the main indication for 965 legal abortions was "psychosomatic exhaustion of the woman caused by alcoholism of the male."

It is perhaps trite to point out that whether or not social and socioeconomic conditions should be allowed to act as indications for abortion is not an empirical question, and cannot be solved by either systematic observation or logical argument. Aleck Bourne, shortly after having made English legal history in the celebrated case of *Rex v. Bourne* by letting it be known that he had aborted a 13-year-old girl who had been raped, observed:[7]

> There is no ultimate appeal or norm beside which a system or detail of ethics can be compared, and therefore we must begin the moral consideration of this subject, abortion, as of all other problems of morality, by remembering that what is rightness or wrongness is the result of the public opinion of the race, epoch, and civilisation as formed by the stress of all other moral considerations which operate on it. The morality of a people is the line of conduct which is found most compatible with the success of the gregarious life, and is the result of adjustment of conflicting individual desires.

It is of interest to observe that world population trends which caused Bourne to oppose relaxing abortion laws in 1939, caused Baird[3] to advocate relaxation quarter of a century later. For the most part people's views on the advisability of abortion for social indications depend on their value-systems and ideas about what ought to be, and it is not surprising to find that opinions range from the totally dismissive[24] to the wish that "we shall reach the stage when only those with a true affection to pass on to their offspring will propagate their kind, and the sins of the fathers will cease to be visited upon the children."[11]

Fortunately there are a number of problems related to socioeconomic aspects of abortion that can be elucidated by empirical enquiry, and these may be posed as a series of questions:

1. Does the prevalence of induced abortion—both legal and criminal—vary with the socioeconomic status of the woman?

2. What is the effect of relaxation of abortion laws on the socioeconomic status of women applying for an abortion?

3. Does the socioeconomic status of the patient help to determine whether the request for an abortion will be granted?

4. What is the socioeconomic status of children born as a result of requests for abortion being refused?

5. What other social variables, relevant to socioeconomic status, help to determine when abortions are sought?

THE SOCIOECONOMIC STATUS OF WOMEN WHO OBTAIN AN INDUCED ABORTION

The increasing number of surveys in various parts of the world[22] do not lend support to the idea that there is always constant relationship between prevalence of induced abortion and socioeconomic status. This is not only because comprehensive and reliable information is understandably not available for countries with strict laws, but also probably because the ease with which an abortion can in fact be obtained in a country is itself a potent determinant of the social class distribution of women obtaining an abortion. The account that follows will therefore group the various countries according to the ease with which an abortion can be obtained in them.

Table 1

	General Population of Japan (Employed men) (Per cent)	Survey Group of 1382 Induced Abortions (Per cent)
Professional and technical workers	5.2	6.4
Managers and officials	3.1	7.2
Clerical workers	9.8	17.3
Sales workers	8.5	13.7
Farmers, lumbermen, fishermen, and related workers	39.7	12.7
Workers in mines and quarries	1.7	—
Workers in operating transport occupations	2.0	3.5
Craftsmen, production process workers and laborers	27.0	32.0
Service workers	2.7	3.7
Occupation not classifiable or not reported	0.2	1.9
No occupation	—	1.6

Countries Where Abortion is Fairly Easily Obtained

Even in countries such as Hungary that virtually allow abortion on request, criminal abortion has not completely disappeared, possibly because of the relative lack of privacy of the official procedure.[64] The incompleteness of official data on abortion is clearly the most serious stumbling block in trying to discover whether the prevalence of abortion really does vary with socioeconomic status. It is clear that the ideal study would compare the socioeconomic status of all women applying for an abortion in a country with very liberal laws with the census data for socioeconomic status of that country.

Koya and Muramatsu[43] have done this for a series of 1382 induced abortions in married women drawn from three geographical areas within Japan, and compared their results with the 1950 census data. The relative incidence of abortion was shown to be highest in women in the 35-39 year old group, and next highest in the 30-34 year old group. Far fewer of the survey group had had the benefit of higher education than would have been expected from the census data. It was the authors' impression that the group as a whole had a lower socioeconomic status than expected, but they were hampered in this last, crucial assessment by lack of adequate census data.

The analysis of the occupations of the women's husbands is much more interesting, since it suggests that use of abortion may not be related to socioeconomic status in a simple way (Table 1).

The group contained proportionately about twice as many "managers and officials" and "clerical workers" as the general population; also it contained somewhat more craftsmen, sales workers and semiskilled laborers. The proportionate number of farmers, lumbermen, and fishermen was less than one third of the general population, and no workers in mines or quarries were included in the group surveyed.

One possible explanation would be to suppose that place of residence (rural/urban) interacts with socioeconomic status to produce the observed results, so that rates are high in urban, and low in rural areas. It is not possible to test this hypothesis with the data presented because of the method of choosing the sample, but Suzumura et al.[62] mention another Japanese survey which indicated that urban rates were higher than rural rates, and this has been confirmed in two recent Scandinavian surveys.

Intriguing as they are, these results must be interpreted with caution for two reasons. First, Suzumura et al.[62] have recently suggested that even now between a third and a half of abortions are not reported to the authorities; and second, because the series includes only abortions carried out for eugenic reasons, and does not include those carried out on the recommendation of a physician under a different section of the Penal Code. The authors properly point out that people with higher education are more likely to use the latter route to procure their abortion.

In Finland, the official statistics record the number of live births, number of legal abortions and the total number of spontaneous and induced abortions. Kaupilla et al.[36] report that in the city of Tampere over a three-year-period the rate for all abortions is highest in the lowest fourth socioeconomic stratum, while the rate for legal abortions is highest in the third. The number of septic abortions has remained constant since the new abortion law allowed abortion for social indications in 1950, and the authors conclude that the number of criminal abortions in the city is "considerable."

The information concerning the socioeconomic status of women seeking abortions in a given hospital is not of any value unless there are grounds for supposing that all women in the area have to use the hospital in question, and the distribution of socioeconomic status in that population is known and can be compared with that of the consulting women. It is, after all, hardly surprising that hospitals in lower class areas have mainly lower class patients.

Kolstad[41] reports on a series of 968 applications for abortion from Drammen Hospital, Norway, which draws patients from an area said to be representative of the Norwegian population, and for which census data are available. Abortions can be carried out for social conditions providing that these can be shown to influence the woman's health. The applicants were shown to be more likely to come from towns and densely populated areas than rural areas. Normative data on the occupational structure of the country were less reliable, but it was shown that workers and artisans were over-represented, and farmers under-represented, in those applying for abortions. Those who did come from rural areas tended to be laborers and foresters, so the data agree fairly well with the Japanese data already quoted.

An altogether different approach is to carry out an interview survey of women of reproductive age in the population, instead of relying on hospital records. Armijo and Monreal[1,2] approached 1860 women drawn on the basis of a probability sample of census information in Santiago, Chile and found that 46 per cent report an abortion in the past, and 26 per cent admit at least one induced abortion. Although abortion is illegal in Chile, the figures are so high that it seems reasonable to include Chile in the group of countries where abortion must be fairly easy to obtain. The abortion rate was highest for women in their twenties in the lower and mid-lower class, with one to three children. The abortions were most often carried out by midwives, amateurs or the women themselves. Only 37 per cent of the women used some means of contraception, and this was much more common in the upper class. The authors conclude that abortion is used as a method of birth control.

Very few of the published surveys of those communist countries where abortion is fairly readily available give information about socioeconomic status, but Verbenko et al.[65] give information on educational status in a survey of 13,500 abortions carried out in the U.S.S.R. in 1962. The authors do not give information about their sampling procedures, and it is not possible to tell what proportion of their subjects fell into the various educational groups. Their results show clearly that only 4.5 per cent of the women with higher education had "non-hospitalised artificial abortions," compared with 15.4 per cent of the poorly educated women. Women had recourse to this latter type of abortion when the law prohibited the operation because they were beyond the twelfth week, when they feared publicity or found the prospect of hospitilization inconvenient.

All the surveys quoted in this section support the view that where abortion is fairly readily available it will be used more frequently by those in the lower socioeconomic levels. This is an unexciting conclusion, since one would of course expect that if abortion is allowed for social indications, it will be more frequent among those who live in poor social conditions. It remains to be seen whether these findings hold good in other settings.

Countries Where Abortion Can Only Be Obtained With Difficulty

In the United States, where the laws relating to abortion are relatively strict, attitudes toward abortion are more liberal and legal abortion is more often used in the upper socioeconomic groups. A recent Gallup Poll[20] of 1511 American adults questioned in November, 1969 asked whether the respondent would favor a law that permitted a woman to go to her doctor to end pregnancy at any time in the first three months. Such a law would be favored by 58 per cent of those with a college education, by 37 per cent of those with a high school education, and only by 31 per cent of those with a grade school education.

Writing from a sociological standpoint, Mechanic[48] views psychiatric indications for abortion as a "backdoor solution" that has come into being because society as a whole is unwilling to liberalize the laws ". . . the unfortunate consequence of this 'backdoor solution' is to discriminate against those who are poor and unsophisticated. The high income and more sophisticated person is more likely to have access to psychiatrists and assistance in dealing with this problem."

There is a good deal of evidence for this assertion within the United States.[23,28,34,45] Gold et al.[23] studied the induced abortions in New York City between 1950 and 1962, and expressed them as rates per 10,000 live births. It will be seen that with descending social status of the type of hospital there are fewer abortions carried out:

	Abortions/ 10,000 Live Births
Proprietary Hospitals	41.6
Private Ward, Voluntary Hospitals	25.6
General Ward, Voluntary Hospitals	7.4
Municipal Hospitals	2.4

Since the socioeconomic status of whites in New York City tends to be superior to that of Puerto Ricans and nonwhites, it is also of interest to note that the percentage of all puerperal deaths due to abortion is only 25.2 per cent for whites, as against 49.4 per cent for nonwhites and 55.6 per cent for Puerto Ricans.

Hall[28] has confirmed these findings at the Sloane Hospital, New York City, by showing that on the private wards there is one abortion on psychiatric grounds per 104 live births, while on the general ward the ratio is 1:1,149. Fifty-three per cent of the private abortions were for psychiatric reasons as against 19 per cent of the ward abortions. He confirms the tendency for more abortions to be carried out on private patients by a questionnaire survey of 65 major U.S. hospitals. This also shows that there are differences between public and private wards in the matter of sterilization since the average parity of ward patients is 6.1 and private patients 3.8.

No one really knows how many criminal abortions there are in the United States, and estimates vary widely.[4,30] Harter and Beasley,[30] for example, argue that since there were only 120 septic abortions per 10,000 live births with only two abortion deaths in New Orleans in the year prior to their paper, that either the women are not having very many induced abortions or they are performed by highly competent abortionists. The authors favor the first alternative, but there are of course others—for example, the number of deaths may be underreported since the death is recorded under some other heading, or many abortions may take place under antibiotic cover. To the extent that septic abortions do provide information about criminal abortions, it is of interest that in his analysis of 223 septic abortion deaths in California, Fox[18] showed that the typical victim comes from a low income group, is aged 25–29, is from a densely populated area and having her first abortion after a number of pregnancies. It would of course be absurd to argue from this that most women having illegal abortions are from low income groups, since it seems more likely that all this survey indicates is that those least able to pay are most likely to get infected.

Kinsey[39] administered a peppery rebuke to those who attempted to discover the incidence of illegal abortion from official data:

> I know of no more untrustworthy fashion of securing statistics on the incidence of any illicit activity than to take official figures that are obtained either through police departments or through reports that are required by state law . . . the number of premarital copulations occurring in a city such as New York is not to be determined by calculating the number of arrests that are made in any year for premarital intercourse. In no type of sexual activity can you begin to get, through official statistics, any approximation of the incidence of behavior—if it is illicit behavior.

Table 2

Years of Education	Total Females (up to age 35)		Females with Premarital Coitus (up to age 35)	
	Premarital Conceptions	Induced Abortions	Premarital Conceptions	Induced Abortions
Grade School (0 - 8 years)	–	6.0%	–	–
High School (9 - 12 years)	11.2%	8.2%	29.7%	21.8%
College (13 - 16 years)	9.8%	8.2%	21.0%	17.6%
Postgraduate (17 years or more)	9.4%	7.9%	19.8%	16.7%

Kinsey's work is based on lengthy and comprehensive interviews with 5293 white and 572 black American women carried out between 1940 and 1949. Unfortunately the sample was in no sense a probability sample of American women, and nearly half the interviews were with college students. Low educational status was under-represented, and the sample as a whole had fewer live births when compared with U.S. census data, and nearly all the respondents lived in urban areas. Educational level attained was used as an index of socioeconomic status, and no distinction was made between legal and illegal induced abortions. It is interesting to see that he finds the incidence of induced abortion only slightly higher in married women than in single women who have had coitus (21.5 per cent to 20.7 per cent), but the incidence is only 9.3 per cent among all single women in the sample. He found that 87 per cent of all abortions were carried out by physicians and only 8 per cent were self-induced.

Premarital conceptions were shown to be more common among the less well-educated, but the same gradient was not nearly so marked when induced abortions were considered. It can be seen from Table 2 that although fewer of the well-educated women who had had coitus had induced abortions when compared with the high school group, in fact the well-educated woman was much less likely to become premaritally pregnant in the first place.

Table 3.—Pregnancies Ending in Induced Abortion

Years of Education	Premarital		Marital	
	White	Black	White	Black
Elementary School (0 - 8 years)	–	18.9%	22.1%	10.0%
High School (9 - 12 years)	63.3%	24.7%	16.3%	7.5%
College (13 - 16 years)	81.7%		17.7%	
Postgraduate (17 years or more)	82.9%	81.2%	15.4%	19.6%

Indeed, if the figures are reexpressed as outcomes of pregnancy, it can be seen that, once she is pregnant, the well-educated girl is very much more likely to end the pregnancy with an induced abortion. This relationship seems to hold good for both whites and blacks with premarital pregnancies, but it no longer holds good for pregnancies that occur within marriages (Table 3).

Hall[27] carried out home interviews with 500 randomly selected women of reproductive age in Lima, Peru, and obtained results that are in striking contrast with those already reported for Santiago in the previous section. The overall abortion rate was only 17 per cent (compared with 46 per cent in Santiago), and only 4 per cent admitted an induced abortion (compared with 26 per cent in Santiago, and 20-22 per cent in U.S.A.). Moreover, the social class gradient observed in Santiago was if anything reversed, since the rate for all abortions was upper level 19 per cent, middle level 20 per cent and lower level 15 per cent. It is possible that her results reflect a true difference between the two cities, since as she says, Lima has a more traditional and conservative background than most other Latin American cities, and the women themselves face up to a four year term of imprisonment if the abortion comes to the notice of the authorities. Her results might therefore support the hypothesis that if abortion is difficult to obtain, the more likely it is to be commoner in the upper socioeconomic levels. On the other hand, the stiff penalties and conservative attitudes might equally have made her subjects defensive and produced spuriously low results. Her interviewers were experienced social workers carrying official letters from the Dean of the Medical School, and this may well have produced relatively greater defensiveness among the lower level women, since they might perceive themselves to be at a great social distance from the interviewer. For all Kinsey's confidence, interview surveys on this topic can be treacherous. While conducting a survey of women known to have had abortions in 1940 Hamilton[29] made the astute observation that:

> The difficulties in arriving at a correct appraisal of circumstances surrounding the abortion do not stop when the momentous question 'induced or spontaneous' is answered. Intentional deception, unintentional misinterpretation and candid truth-telling mingle in varying proportions in the mass response to each question. Many of the answers undoubtedly represent the patient's idea of what *ought* to be the case and are a half-conscious attempt to deceive not only the investigator, but herself as well.

Hamilton herself studied 527 consecutive admissions for termination of pregnancy to Bellevue Hospital, New York, and aimed to divide them into definitely induced abortions, definitely spontaneous, and various intermediate groups with a view to comparing the social conditions of the induced abortions with a control group of spontaneous abortions. No significant differences were found between the groups for socioeconomic status, but this may have been because the majority of the patients had very bad housing conditions and were very poor, so that there was insufficient variation on these dimensions within her groups. But as she was well aware, the most serious methodological flaw in her design—and indeed, in any design based on interview data—was whether one could believe the patient's claim that their abortion was spontaneous: "Two, who were most persistent in their denial (of induction), in terminal delirium described their experience with the abortionist."[29] Fortunately, very few research workers have this opportunity of really finding out about abortion.

The position regarding abortion in the United States can be summarized by saying that there is good evidence for supposing that legal abortions are more common in higher socioeconomic groups, and also that incompetently performed illegal abortions resulting in sepsis and death are more common in lower socioeconomic groups. There is no very solid evidence for supposing that there is a social class gradient for *all* illegal abortions, although common sense suggests that when carried out by a physician in a private nursing home they are more common among the rich, since the procedure is known to be fairly expensive.[63] Indeed, it seems probable that each social class has its own accepted ways of dealing with an unwanted pregnancy: jet travel to a country with liberal laws or "psychiatric" indications for the rich, and a cheaper local abortionist or self-induced methods for the poor.

The Situation in Sweden

The situation in Sweden is intermediate between the two groups of countries described above since although abortions are permitted for psychiatric and "extended medical" indications, the application procedure is fairly involved and refusals are quite common. Höök[32] showed that the occupational status of the male partners of 294 women whose application for abortion on psychiatric grounds was refused was in close agreement with the general population as shown in the 1948 election statistics. She also showed that the socioeconomic status of the male partners in her groups of refused women was similar to that found by Ekblad[13] in his group of 479 women whose application was granted.

These findings must be interpreted with considerable reserve, since they apply only to the population of women who apply through official channels for a termination on psychiatric grounds, and also, as Höök observes:

> As a general equalisation of the economic differences between the social classes has taken place in the past few decades a division of women into different socioeconomic groups would seem to be of limited value . . . No appreciable differences in the manner of living between the different classes in the material could be noted. Any differences that were observable were more in the nature of family traditions and social identification.

None of the countries discussed in the preceding two sections could really claim this degree of economic equality. It is, however, legitimate to make two observations about these findings. First, in this cultural setting there is no evidence that women applying for an official abortion are more likely to come from any particular socioeconomic stratum of the population. Second, if socioeconomic factors were taken into account in making the decision whether or not to abort, one would have expected that Ekblad's series of granted abortions should have come from lower socioeconomic strata than Höök's series of refused abortions, but it appears that this is not the case.

THE EFFECT OF RELAXING THE ABORTION LAWS ON THE SOCIOECONOMIC STATUS OF WOMEN APPLYING FOR ABORTION

Three recent surveys in different countries review the effects of a relaxation of the abortion laws, and include data on socioeconomic status in their findings. Diggory[12] reports a personal series of 1000 abortions carried out since the new English Abortion Act and compares their socioeconomic status with census data both for the locality and the whole country (Table 4).

It can be seen that social classes I and II are relatively over-represented, and III and IV under-represented, among those availing themselves of an abortion under the new law.

Heller and Whittington[31] report on their early experience with a more liberal abortion law in the state of Colorado, and note that despite a great increase in the number of abortions now being carried out the lowest socioeconomic class does not seem to be availing itself of the new facilities.

Kaupilla et al[36] compare the abortions carried out in a Finnish city during two three year periods, before and after liberalization of the law. Although the rate for all induced abortions is highest in the lowest socioeconomic group, in the latter period the greatest number of legal abortions was being carried out in the third rather than the lowest socioeconomic stratum.

Although socioeconomic status was measured in a different way in each of these three studies, taken together they suggest that there is a reluctance to use a new service among lower income people that could be called "social viscosity." It is not possible to say from these data whether this is because there is a slowness in finding out about and using a new service, or whether there is a more enduring relationship between socioeconomic factors and seeking social care. Two studies in a related field suggest that both components may play a part.

Richardson[55] reports on the first year of operation of an experimental program to enable pregnant schoolgirls to continue their education during pregnancy. Her study compares an index group of 109 girls who had attended the program with 123 girls who were eligible but were not enrolled. The girls in the index group were from a higher socioeconomic group than the

Table 4.—Abortions by Social Class

Locality	Social Class				
	I	II	III	IV	V
Abortion Series (N=1000)	5.5%	41.2%	34.7%	10.8%	7.5%
London and S.E. England (1961 census)	1.1%	15.0%	48.6%	24.4%	6.6%
England and Wales (1966 census)	0.8%	15.3%	46.7%	28.5%	7.5%

controls, and the author speculates that "increased income is associated with more awareness of facilities available in the community and knowledge about obtaining services." Bernstein and Sauber[5] report on the medical and social antenatal care obtained by 520 unmarried mothers in New York, and showed that those with higher education were both more likely to obtain medical antenatal care early in the pregnancy, and to seek help from social services. Women with only a grade school education were not only less likely to have had contact with social agencies than college girls, but if they did have contact it was far more likely to be a minimal contact with a clinic social worker or bureau of public assistance official. In contrast the better educated were more likely to know about and use a range of services from social agencies.

The attempt to explain the survey findings reported in this section in terms of "social viscosity" assumes that social factors have their effects on the behavior of the pregnant woman, rather than on the doctor whom she consults. It would have been possible, for example, for the doctors themselves to have been responsible for the observed results by being less likely to agree to abortions among women of lower socioeconomic status. The next section therefore examines the behavior of the doctors themselves.

The Effect of Socioeconomic Status in Determining Whether a Request for Abortion is Granted

A number of recently published studies compare the social characteristics of patients whose requests for an abortion have been granted with those for the patients whose request was refused.[10,31,37,54] It might at first sight seem that these studies would allow one to say what the social indications for abortion really are, but on reflection it is clear that while they serve as a valuable record of what their authors actually do, they cannot possibly give any indication about what ought to be, and indeed seem destined to become curiosities for future historians of social medicine. One can say, for example, that Clark et al.[10] are less likely to terminate a patient who is a young, single girl with illegitimate children and more likely to do so if she is older, married, and has at least two legitimate children: whether or not she has emotional support available will not sway them either way. Kenyon[37] on the other hand, is more likely to refuse a patient if she is single, has a superior intelligence and was educated beyond the age of 15, and more likely to agree if she is married and strikes him as being a suicidal risk. Neither of these investigators mentions socioeconomic status of their two groups, but Clark et al. mention that 81 of their 229 patients followed up had asked for abortion because of "bad social conditions"; of these, 47 were terminated and 34 refused.

If psychiatrists really were swayed by bad social conditions in making their recommendations for termination, then it would be reasonable to expect that the socioeconomic status of patients whose application is accepted would be worse than the group who are refused. Although factual information is exiguous, there is some reason to suppose that this is not so. It has already been shown that the socioeconomic status of both Höök's[32] and Ekblad's[13]

Swedish studies did not differ from the Swedish general population, and Heller and Whittington's[31] series of 109 approved and 59 rejected abortion applications in Denver, Colorado gives detailed information about socio-economic status. If their two groups of patients are divided into four income groups, then it can be seen that while abortions seem more likely to be approved in the midincome range ($4000–8000) relative to either extreme, in fact the difference between the two distributions is not significant (chi square=4.34 on 3 d.f., reviewer's calculation). There is therefore no evidence in the available data to support the idea that socioeconomic status of patients who are granted a legal abortion is any different from those who are refused.

Deacon[11] has observed, from the gynecologist's standpoint, that a psychiatrist's opinion on termination: ". . . will inevitably depend on the sympathy that his colleague feels for the plight of the applicant." If this is so, then it would seem to be sympathy for the sorts of plight that can occur equally well in upper and in lower strata of society.

The Socioeconomic Status of Children Born as a Result of Requests for Abortion Being Refused

Forssman and Thuwe[17] studied a group of 197 women who were refused legal abortion in Goetborg, Sweden between 1939 and 1941. A total of 120 children survived into adult life as a result of the refusal to abort, and this group was compared with a control group chosen by taking the next child of the same sex in the hospital birth register after each index child. The socioeconomic status of the two groups at birth was found to be similar—with the proviso that where an index child was adopted it was assigned the socio-economic status of the adopting parents. The two groups of children were followed up until their twenty-first birthday.

Many more of the unwanted (index) children had not had a secure family life in childhood. They were registered more often in psychiatric services, for antisocial and criminal behavior, and for public assistance. Far fewer had had education beyond the obligatory age, and more were educationally subnormal. More of the females married early and had children early. Thus, the very fact that a woman seeks an authorized abortion, no matter how trivial her grounds may appear to some, means that the expected child will have to surmount greater social and mental handicaps than its peers, and will run a greater risk of an inferior standing in life. In the author's opinion (and, indeed, in the reviewer's opinion) legislation on abortion should also take account of the social risks to which the expected child will be exposed.

Social Variables Relevant to Socioeconomic Status that Help Determine When Abortions Are Sought

If every married woman felt her family budget sufficient to provide satisfactorily for unlimited children, if there were no social stigma associated with illegitimacy, the incidence of induced abortion would, no doubt, be reduced to a fraction of its present magnitude. The relative nature of economic and social pressure must be

stressed. An income which would seem ample for four children to a woman ac
customed to one standard of living would seem to another hopelessly inadequat
for one. Illegitimacy is accepted in certain social groups with no more than
passing sneer, in others it means ruin to the mother and life-long handicap to th
child.[29]

In the thirty years since Hamilton wrote these words, legal abortion ha
been introduced in Japan and Eastern Europe for all of these social indica
tions—too large a family, economic hardship and illegitimacy. Since size o
family is obviously relevant to socioeconomic status, it remains to explore thi
variable in greater detail.

Tietze[32,63] compared 863 illegal abortions carried out in an eastern city in
the United States with women having babies at home in the same city, anc
found that parity was higher among the women having abortions. He ob
served that abortion was used not as a method of child spacing but of limitin
the ultimate size of the family. Höök confirmed the findings that womer
applying for abortions have more children than the population as a whole.

Miltenyi and Szabady[50] reviewed the effect of legalization of abortion in
Hungary and observed that while there was no reduction in the number of
pregnancies, the number of families with one, two or three children had in
creased, while the number of childless families and families with four or more
children had decreased. They concluded that the number of living children is
the strongest factor which makes married women decide to take advantage
of induced abortion. Use of contraceptives had remained constant at only
20-30 per cent.

Koya et al.[44] produced similar figures for Japan—abortion is more likely
among women in their thirties with two to three live children. Again, only
27 per cent had practiced contraception prior to abortion. Koya[42] has also
noted that abortion is more likely when there is at least one boy as the surviv
ing child or among the surviving children, although with the sample size that
he used this finding did not reach statistical significance.

In Santiago, Chile, Requena[57] studied 448 women of reproductive age
divided into two groups: those that used contraceptives and those that used
abortion as their method of birth control. Only 20 per cent used contraceptives,
and only 5 per cent used effective methods such as the condom. The more
educated women were more likely to use contraception than the illiterates,
while abortion did not seem to relate to level of education. Religion—Catholic
versus "other" and "none"—seemed to make very little difference to what the
women actually did. Use of abortion became much more common with
advancing age, but use of contraception was independent of age. Abortion
was much more common with advancing family size, so that with four or
more children, 57 per cent used abortion as against 20 per cent using contraception. There was no difference for white-collar workers, but among
manual laborers and housewives twice as many used abortion as used contraception. Although contraceptives were offered to all the women who did not
use them, only 56 per cent availed themselves of the offer.

These findings have been given at some length since although to most doctors abortion is an event with complex medical and psychiatric indications, to women in many parts of the world it is merely an uncomfortable and dangerous form of birth control.

It must not be assumed that the prevalence of abortion in various socio-economic levels necessarily reflects the need for abortion at that level. Muller[51] has argued that in lower socioeconomic levels there is a greater need for abortions, although they are in fact more difficult to obtain through legal channels. She supports this by noting that "low-income couples express the same family size goals as higher income couples, but are less successful, on the whole, in the use of contraception."[35] The outcome of present United States abortion policies is to increase the number of unwanted children in the lower socioeconomic strata, and with them the associated problems of neglect, delinquency and social incapacity for the care of children.[51]

Sometimes a woman is granted an abortion on social grounds on condition that she accepts sterilization as well. Such blackmailing tactics are even less justifiable in the light of Ekblad's findings[14,15] on the prognosis of childless women after sterilization. Over half of the 60 patients were dissatisfied with the sterilization and regretted it, and the vast majority of these patients experienced an unsatisfied longing for children. One third of the group had become depressed and nervous since the operation. The greater the psychiatric indications for sterilization, the greater the risk of adverse mental after-effects. At greatest risk were girls of subnormal intelligence who were sterilized on eugenic grounds as a condition for the abortion. Ekblad argues the case for considering the merits of abortion and sterilization separately, and exercising considerable restraint in assigning eugenic grounds especially if there is any doubt in the matter. Fairly similar findings are reported from London by McCoy.[47]

Baird[3] deals with women who seek an abortion after having had three or four children by encouraging them to have the child, but to have a sterilization after the delivery. The results of this policy are that women in lower social classes are more likely to be dealt with in this way, while women of upper classes are more likely to be granted an abortion, often on psychiatric grounds. This is shown in Table 5.

Table 5

Operation	I–II	Social Class III	IV–V	Number of Cases
Curettage or hysterotomy unmarried	54%	33%	4%	24
Curettage, married	33%	39%	20%	39
Hysterotomy and tubal ligation	15%	45%	37%	137
Post partum tubal ligation	9%	48%	43%	413
All Aberdeen	14%	59%	27%	

Baird justifies this by observing:

> Women in low socio-economic groups are less accustomed to long term plan-
> ning . . . . by the time three of four children have arrived in quick succession they
> may find themselves in a local authority house, but possibly unable to cope physically
> and financially with the situation. Some ask to have the pregnancy terminated, but
> more often they agree to continue with it so long as they have the promise of an
> operation for tubal ligation in the puerperium. The assurance that the current
> pregnancy will be the last makes it possible for many to accept the situation.[3]

Summary

Although precedents can be found in the literature for a very wide range of
social events being used to justify abortion, this only tells us what individual
doctors have done, not what they ought to have done, or what is desirable.
Nonetheless empirical research has provided information that is of some assistance in weighing up the pros and cons of an individual case. From the
woman's point of view, Höök[32] has shown that only 23 per cent of her series
of women refused abortion accepted the pregnancy and made a good adjustment: a further 53 per cent adjusted themselves eventually after a "variety
of insufficiency reactions" in the first 18 months, while no fewer than 24 per
cent had adjusted so poorly to the situation that they still had symptoms that
were present at follow-up about 10 years later. Patients who were less than 26
years old, unmarried and with deviating personalities were especially likely
to adjust poorly to the situation. It is disconcerting to remember that young
unmarried women are more likely to be refused in the two English surveys
reported earlier.[10,37] From the unborn child's point of view, we have seen that
the child can expect greater social and mental handicaps if he comes into the
world, and that the outcome of restrictive abortion policies is to produce more
unwanted children among lower socioeconomic groups.

A final point concerns who should make such social recommendations for
abortion, if they are to be made at all. Psychiatrists, as an obstetrician un-
kindly pointed out,[26] do not have a monopoly of human understanding, and
such assessments might equally be made by obstetricians themselves, by
family doctors and by medical social workers.

The majority of abortions in many parts of the world are carried out for
social indications. In countries where abortion is fairly easy to obtain the
available evidence suggests that it is more common among the lower social
classes, and is indeed often used as the method of birth control. In countries
with stricter laws there is much convergent evidence which suggests that
legal abortions are more commonly done in higher socioeconomic groups,
and little to suggest that socioeconomic factors are taken into account in
deciding on a termination for psychiatric grounds.

There is little good evidence concerning the socioeconomic distribution of
illegal abortions in these countries, although one study suggests that once a
single girl is pregnant, she is more likely to obtain an abortion if she has had
a college education. Indirect evidence suggests that restrictive abortion laws
increase the number of unwanted children among lower social classes. The

adverse psychological effects of refusing an application for abortion are described, and there is some evidence that those who are most at risk are most likely to be refused. The babies that are born as a result of refusing an application for abortion are shown to be at a disadvantage both socially and psychologically.

ACKNOWLEDGMENTS

My thanks are due to Dr. R. Bruce Sloane, who provided consistent encouragement and the facilities for carrying out this research. Dr. A. Jablensky, Mr. M. P. Lippner, Dr. Leon Sherashefsky, Miss K. Spraggins, Dr. R. Tislow and Dr. R. Vispo very kindly provided translations of papers in Serbo-Croat, Czech, Russian, Spanish and German. Miss Judy Lin and the reference librarians at Temple Medical School Library made everything possible by repeatedly tracking down articles in obscure journals at short notice.

REFERENCES

1. Armijo, R., and Monreal, T.: Epidemiologia del aborto provocado en Santiago, Chile. Rev. Med. Chile. 92:548-557, 1964.

2. —, and —: El problema del aborto provocado en Chile. Rev. Med. Chile. 93: 357-362, 1965.

3. Baird, D.: A fifth freedom. Brit. Med. J. 2:1141-1148, 1965.

4. Barno, A.: Criminal abortion—deaths and suicide in pregnancy in Minnesota (1950-1964). Minn. Med. 50:11-16, 1967.

5. Bernstein, B., and Sauber, M.: Deterrents to early prenatal care and social services among women pregnant out-of-wedlock. New York State Dept. of Welfare, Albany, New York, 1960.

6. Bolter, S.: The psychiatrist's role in therapeutic abortion: the unwitting accomplice. Am. J. Psychiatry. 119:312, 1962.

7. Bourne, A.: Some social aspects of abortion. (Trans. Obst. Soc.). Edinburgh Med. J. 105-124, May, 1939.

8. Calderone, M. S.: Abortion in the United States. New York, Harper and Hoeber, 1958.

9. Chroscielewski, E., and Simm, S.: L'aspect social et medico-social du probleme de la regulation des naissances en Pologne. Ann. Med. Leg. 47:527-532, 1967.

10. Clark, M., Forstner, I., Pond, P.A., and Tredgold, R. F.: Sequels of unwanted pregnancy. Lancet 2:501-503, 1968.

11. Deacon, A. L.: Sequels of unwanted pregnancy. Lancet 2:730, 1968.

12. Diggory, P. L. C.: Some experiences of therapeutic abortion. Lancet 873-875, 1969.

13. Ekblad, M.: Induced abortion on psychiatric grounds. Acta Psych. Scand. Suppl. 99, 1955.

14. —: The prognosis after sterilization on social psychiatric grounds. Acta Psych. Scand. Suppl. 161, 1961.

15. —: Social psychiatric prognosis after sterilization of women without children. A follow-up of 60 women. Acta Psych. Scand. 39:481-514, 1963.

16. Faraj, E.: Aborto Factores Medico Sociales. Rev. Med. Hondur. 33:157-163, 1963.

17. Forssman, H., and Thuwe, I.: 120 children born after application for therapeutic abortion refused. (Their mental health, social adjustment and educational level up to the age of 21). Acta Psych. Scand. 42: 71-88, 1966.

18. Fox, L. P.: Abortion deaths. Amer. J. Obstet. Gynec. 98:645, 1967.

19. Fox, R.: The law on abortion. Lancet 1:542, 1966.

20. Gallup Poll: 40% believe abortion should be a legal right. Washington Post. p. A6, Sunday, Nov. 30, 1969.

21. Gebhard, P., Pomeroy, W., Martin, C. and Christenson, C.: Pregnancy, Birth and Abortion. New York, Harper and Hoeber, 1958.

22. afGeijerstam, G. K.: An annotated bibliography of induced abortion. University of Michigan, 1969.

23. Gold, E., Erhardt, C. L., Jacobziner, H., and Nelson, F. G.: Therapeutic abortions in New York City: A 20 year review. Amer. J. Pub. Health. 55:964, 1965.

24. Gordon, H.: Genetical, social and medical aspects of abortion. S. Afr. Med. J. 42:721-730, 1968.

25. Guttmacher, A. F.: The shrinking non-psychiatric indications for abortion. *In*

Rosen, H. (Ed.): Abortion in America. New York, Beacon Press, 1954, pp. 12–21.

26. Haldane, F. P.: Sequels of unwanted pregnancy. Lancet 2:678-679, 1968.

27. Hall, M. F.: Birth control in Lima, Peru—attitudes and practices. Milbank Mem. Fund Quart. 43:409, 1965.

28. Hall, R. E.: Therapeutic abortion, sterilization and contraception. Amer. J. Obstet. Gynec. 91:518, 1965.

29. Hamilton, V. C.: Some sociological and psychological observations on abortion. Amer. J. Obstet. Gynec. 39:919-928, 1940.

30. Harter, C. L., and Beasley, J. D.: A survey concerning induced abortions in New Orleans. Amer. J. Pub. Health. 57:1937, 1967.

31. Heller A., and Whittington, H. G.: The Colorado story: Denver General Hospital experience with the change in the law on therapeutic abortion. Amer. J. Psychiat. 125:809-816, 1968.

32. Höök, K.: Refused abortion—A follow-up study of 249 women. Acta Psychiat. Scand. Suppl. 168. Vol. 39, 1963.

33. Ingman, O.: On the influence of alcohol abuse of the husband on the indications for abortion. Ann. Chir. Gynaec. Fenn. 55:301, 1966.

34. Ingram, J. M.: Interruption of pregnancy for psychiatric indication—a suggested method of control. Obstet. Gynec. 29:251, 1967.

35. Jaffe, F. S., and Guttmacher, A.: Family planning programs in the United States. Demography Vol. 5, No. 2, p. 1, 1968.

36. Kauppila, O., Aro, P., and Soiza, K.: The effect of the Abortion Act of 1950 on abortions—in the city of Tampere. Duodecim 78:956, 1962.

37. Kenyon, F. E.: Termination of pregnancy on psychiatric grounds: a comparative study of 61 cases. Brit. J. Med. Psychol. 42:243-254, 1969.

38. Kinsey, A. C.: In Calderone, M. (Ed.): Abortion in the United States. New York, Harper and Hoeber, 1958.

39. —: Illegal abortion in the United States. In Roberts, R. W. (Ed.). The Unwed Mother. New York, Harper and Row, pp. 191-200, 1966.

40. Kolarova, O., and Gruber, A.: Problems of artificial interruption of pregnancy of Southern Moravia. Demografie 7: 154, 1965.

41. Kolstad, P.: Therapeutic abortion: A clinical study based upon 968 cases from a Norwegian hospital, 1940-1953. Acta Obstet. Gynec. Scand. Vol. 36, Suppl. 6, 1957.

42. Koya, Y.: Induced abortion in Japan. Milbank Mem. Fund Quart. 32:282-293, 1954.

43. Koya, T., and Muramatsu, M.: A survey of health and demographic aspects of induced abortion in Japan. Report No. 2. Bull. Inst. Pub. Health of Japan. 3:18–24, 1954.

44. Koya, Y., Agota, S., and Koya, T.: A study of induced abortion in Japan and its significance. Asian Med. J. 8:265, 1965.

45. Kummer, J. M., and Leavy, Z.: Therapeutic abortion law confusion. JAMA 195:96, 1966.

46. Lidz, T.: In Calderone, M. (Ed.): Abortion in the United States. New York, Harper and Hoeber, 1958, p. 141.

47. McCoy, D. R.: The emotional reactions of women to therapeutic abortion and sterilisation. J. Obstet. Gynaec. Brit. Comm. 75:1054-1057, 1968.

48. Mechanic, D.: Medical sociology—A selective view. New York, The Free Press, 1968, p. 381.

49. Miltenyi, K.: Social and psychological factors affecting fertility in a legalized abortion system. Proc. World Pop. Conf. 1965. 2:318. New York, United Nations, 1967.

50. —, and Szabady, E.: The problem of abortion in Hungary: demographic and health aspects. Demografie 7:303, 1964.

51. Muller, C.: Socio-economic outcomes of present abortion policy. Paper delivered at the workshop on abortion, N.I.M.H., Washington, December 15, 1969.

52. Muramatsu, M., and Ogino, H.: Estimation of the total numbers of induced abortions as well as of sterilizations for females in Japan in 1952 and 1953. Bull. Inst. Pub. Health of Japan. 4:10-11, 1954.

53. Olki, M.: The situation of abortion in Finland. E. Mehlan, K-H. Leipzig, Georg Thieme, 1961.

54. Rauramo, L., and Gronroos, M.: Subjective and objective motivation for legal abortion at a social advice center. Ann. Chir. Gynaec. Fenn. 49:1, 1960.

55. Richardson, A.: Evaluation of a public school program for pregnant girls. Bureau of Social Science Research, Inc., Washington, D.C., 1966.

56. Roemer, R.: Abortion law: the ap-

proaches of different nations. Amer. J. Pub. Health. 57:1906, 1967.

57. Requena, M.: Studies of family planning in the Quinta Normal District of Santiago. Milbank Mem. Fund Quart. 43:69, 1965.

58. Rosen, H.: Abortion in America. New York, Beacon Press, 1954.

59. —: In Calderone, M. (Ed.): Abortion in the United States. New York, Harper and Hoeber, 1958, p. 141.

60. Sim, M.: Abortion and the psychiatrist. Brit. Med. J. 2:145-148, 1963.

61. Sloane, R. B.: The unwanted pregnancy. New Eng. J. Med. 280:1206, 1969.

62. Suzumura, M., and Kikuchi, S.: Induced abortion in Japan—review of the literature. J. Jap. Obstet. Gynaec. Soc. 13:179-197, 1966.

63. Tietze, C.: Report on a series of illegal abortions induced by physicians. Hum. Biol. 21:60, 1949.

64. —: Abortion in Europe. Am. J. Pub. Health. 57:1923, 1967.

65. Verbenko, A. A., Il'in, S. E., Chusova, V. N., and Al'shevskaya, T. N.: Concerning the social-hygienic meaning of abortion. Zdravoskhr. Ross. Fed. 10:22-26, 1966.

66. Vojta, M.: New significance of abortion and interruption of pregnancy for the development of the population. S. R. B. ed. Demograficky Sbornik, 1961.

Therapeutic Abortion in Great Britain

By D. A. POND, M.D., F.R.C.P., D.P.M.

A LTHOUGH THE NEW ACT governing therapeutic termination of pregnancy has been in operation a little over a year, some facts and figures about the effects are becoming available.[4,9] The Act, which requires a record of all terminations done to be sent to the Department of Health and Social Security (the former Ministry of Health), assures for the first time fairly accurate figures available on the total number of legal abortions done in this country. Confidentiality of the information sent is ensured by having the form sent to the Chief Medical Officer and not to a lay administrator. Two practitioners (preferably the patient's usual general practitioner and a consultant who is usually the gynecologist intending to operate) certify the need for operation on one or more of the following grounds:

1. The continuance of the pregnancy would involve risk to the life of the pregnant woman greater than if the pregnancy were terminated.

2. The continuance of the pregnancy would involve risk of injury to the physical or mental health of the pregnant woman greater than if the pregnancy were terminated.

3. The continuance of the pregnancy would involve risk of injury to the physical or mental health of existing children of the pregnant woman greater than if the pregnancy were terminated.

4. There is a substantial risk that if the child were born it would suffer from such physical or mental abnormalities as to be seriously handicapped.

In practice, the first and second causes are the ones most commonly given, although in many cases the second cannot be easily distinguished from the third. As Baird[2] has said in this connection, one cannot and should not separate "medical" from "social." Amongst other opinions, advice from medical defense societies has made it clear that adequate evaluaton of a woman's social and psychological situation can rarely be made by a few minutes' interview in a busy and often rather public gynecological outpatient department, and even the general practitioners' reports may need supplementing by social workers' reports, based on home visits if necessary.

As would be expected, the total number of terminations known to be done has gone up by leaps and bounds, and there appears to be no sign as yet of the curve flattering out. The numbers done had in fact started to rise in 1966 and 1967, presumably reflecting more permissive attitudes of gynecologists in anticipation of the new Act. Although all areas of the country are doing more terminations, there are marked and puzzling differences between the rates in the national health hospitals of one area and another, with parts of London having easily the highest rate (6.5 per 1000 women aged 15 to 49 years). Most regions have rates between 2 and 3 per 1000, but Liverpool has a rate of 1.1 per 1000. In the areas of the highest national health service rates, up to 40 per cent of the terminations have been done privately; that is to say, not free under the National Health Service, but in private nursing homes which have been specifically approved and registered for this purpose. The Registrar General's figures show that practically all these private abortions are done in the northwest region of London, which includes the Harley Street area. It is also of interest that 70 per cent of the women terminated in these approved nursing homes were single, whereas the percentage in national health service hospitals all over the country varied between 22 per cent and 37 per cent with the exception of the London Teaching Hospital where the percentage was 47 per cent, exactly the same as the proportion over the whole of Britain. Furthermore, the proportion of the women terminated who were nulliparous was 66 per cent in the Northwest Metropolitan Region (including both national health service and approved nursing home places) whereas in the rest of the country the proportion varied between 22 per cent and 38 per cent with the London teaching hospitals rather higher at 43 per cent. Thus, the capital seems to be more "permissive" as regards terminations both in the health service hospitals and privately.

The existence of this large private sector strongly suggests that at any rate in some areas of the country many requests for termination under the health service are being turned down and then referred elsewhere. Privately organized and financed pregnancy advisory services are being started in several areas in response to this need. They are, of course, operating publicly and within the law as it stands at present. The Minister of Health has gone on record as rightly being concerned about the movement of women to the bigger cities, and especially London, for terminations that have been refused locally. This is undoubtedly much more important numerically and socially than the notoriety enjoyed briefly by reports of plane loads of women coming from abroad for cheap and easy terminations on demand (only relatively cheap of course, as none of these patients can be treated under the national health service).

The increased number of operations has given rise to claims and counterclaims that gynecological wards and operating theaters are being overloaded and that waiting lists for serious conditions, such as cancer, are lengthening. Hard facts about waiting lists are difficult to come by; for what it is worth the annual statistical returns for the whole country in fact show a very small fall in those waiting (for the second year running), but all sorts of factors enter into this calculation. To meet the need, the suggestion has several times been made that special "Abortion Clinics" should be set up. There are various possible methods of doing this; for example, they might be staffed by consultant gynecologists on a sessional basis, and perhaps patients might pay on a sliding scale according to their means, though it is unclear why this service should be put on a par with teeth and spectacles as the only areas so far where patients make a specific contribution. In any case, if dangerous arrears of patients on waiting lists are occurring, this is an argument for increasing the gynecological services, not for cutting down the number of terminations.

One has every sympathy with gynecologists who feel that they are often being publicly abused while at the same time expected to do society's dirty work for them. They would be relieved of this role almost completely if and when a simple safe "abortion pill" is discovered which would cleanly and painlessly dissolve the fetus in utero. The real moral and social difficulties will then become clearer—should this pill be freely on sale with the aspirins in drug stores, or available only on doctor's prescription (and inevitably then from the black market as well)?

The increase in the number of terminations is presumably paralleled by a decrease in the number of illegal abortions, though again hard facts on this matter are notoriously difficult to obtain, as has been realized for years in countries such as Sweden and some in Eastern Europe where liberal laws were introduced some time ago.[7] About 100,000 illegal abortions per year has been widely quoted as the best guess for the years preceding the workings of the new Act. However, as Goodhart[6] has pointed out, the known death rate after these operations is about 30 per year, which makes it a remarkably safe procedure. Even if the illegal abortion rate were substantially less than 100,000, it is unlikely to have been close to the current termination rate which is less than half that. Illegal abortions are therefore probably still going on, but at a lower rate, much as had been the experience of Sweden following their new, more liberal abortion law. Godber[5] has pointed out that the number of emergency admissions to hospitals under the London Emergency Beds Scheme has fallen by a third between 1966 and 1969 for treatment after abortion. Even countries with free abortion on demand do not seem to eradicate illegal abortion completely. In Sweden women may be reluctant to put their case to the special Board, or refuse to accept their veto. In some cases one has seen complex psychological disorders—guilt feelings that can only be assuaged by what may be half unconsciously seen as self-mutilation. In a few cases it seems that in fact the catharsis from "doing it yourself" was better than if the patient had had to collude with an authority figure to rid herself of a bad object, though obviously in these cases it would be better still if the patient could work through these fantasies in psychotherapy rather than be exposed to the usual risks of back street abortions.

For many years Sir Dugald Baird[2] and his colleagues in Aberdeen have been quietly carrying out a termination policy similar to that which now obtains in many parts of the country since the new Act, giving a rate of about 4/1000. Yet even in Aberdeen there has been some increase in demand in the past years, though the number of those referred who are refused termination (about half) is unchanged.[1] The increased demand is mainly from younger women, often illegitimately pregnant. The latter now make up half the total done, whereas it used to be about 10 per cent. The fact that the demand from older married women, who have had "enough children," is more or less unchanged, is probably due to the relatively efficient and widespread system of contraceptive advice which has been available for some years in Aberdeen. Tubal ligation is also freely offered to women after multiple pregnancies and is frequently carried out.[2] One cannot, unfortunately, assume that the women (and the doctors) of the rest of the country will emulate solid commonsense Aberdonian behavior in this any more than in many other matters.

The present state of public opinion and medical practice on termination still leave unsettled the crucial issue of who is to make the final decision. Is it to be "abortion on demand" by the client, and no questions asked, or will the doctor be able to have the final say, and if so, which doctor—the general practitioner, the psychiatrist, or the gynecologist—or even perhaps the social worker? With few exceptions most consultants (and especially consultant gynecologists) are solidly against abortion on demand. This may, in part, explain the growth of the facilities for private termination. The combined British Medical Association/Royal College of Obstetricians and Gynecologists' demand for terminations to be done only by consultant gynecologists can be seen as partly a laudable attempt to keep up the standards, but also partly as an effort to restrict the work of these private clinics. The position about abortion amongst gynecologists is thus in marked contrast to their attitude toward sterilization which most of them will now do virtually on demand. It must be the only mutilating procedure thus favored, and with the legal position recently clarified, thanks largely to the activities of the Simon Trust, male sterilization is slowly coming into more general use.

As stated elsewhere[8] termination on demand is practicable and sound psychologically for the older married women who have had "enough" children. Psychiatric sequelae are rare at this age, and with the much more widespread use of better contraceptive methods "mistakes" leading to conception are likely to be genuine. Only occasionally does one come across a compulsive child-bearer at this age. In any case, the correct treatment for such a psychological disturbance is psychotherapy rather than allowing the compulsion to be gratified by more and more children.

The main problems center on the younger and often single woman. It is on this group that the biggest emotional impact is made by those campaigning for more "liberal" laws. The psychological situations of these women are in fact varied. In some there is an unconscious need to become pregnant (or, in the case of a man, an unconscious need to impregnate) in order to prove how, albeit fallaciously, they are capable of full adult sexuality. This is suggested by the astonishing frequency with which couples, who should and do know better, have intercourse without any sort of contraceptive measures being taken. In the University College Hospital series[3] it was reported that about 40 per cent admitted to using no contraceptive: similar proportions have been reported by others. The introduction of a more liberal abortion law without any effort to improve the availability and *use* of family planning methods is likely to result in the sort of chaotic conditions that prevailed in Japan and some eastern European countries for a while, to the disgruntlement of the medical profession and a great deal of unhappiness all round. The Department of Health and Social Security has been energetically prodding local hospitals and clinics to provide more free contraceptive advice under the health service, but progress is pitifully slow. Education is equally important to see that these services are understood and used. This must be directed to young men as well as young women, since the male's role in causing conception is often so surprisingly ignored that one might imagine parthenogenesis was the rule.

It is sometimes asserted that a liberal abortion law results in public indifference to parenthood, less attention to child care, and less "reverence for life."

There is no evidence that this is so, and in many ways there is some evidence to the contrary in the increasing public concern about child welfare. A more responsible attitude would mean that children will be born only into families which are ready and willing to have them. Unfortunately, there is as yet no perceptible fall-off in the number of unwanted children born. Orphanages are still full, and for the first time the number of children available for adoption nears the number of childless families wanting children. One may hope (optimistically perhaps) that better education in sexual behavior and more widespread use of contraception will catch up with people's present behavior so that demands for termination will settle out at a fairly low level. The social revolution needed to ensure proper population control can be separated more and more from what men and women regard as their "right" sexual behavior, thanks to advances in medical knowledge. As usual, every new advance in knowledge brings it own new problem, and doctors especially are experiencing some difficulty in adjusting to their changing roles in society. No longer are physicians virtually the sole arbiters of some aspects of behavior, but members of a team in the social services often making decisions with, and not for, their patients.

SUMMARY

Since 1967 the new Act in Britain permits legal termination of pregnancy where its continuance would involve greater risk to the life of the mother, or to her physical and mental health or to that of her existing children, or if there is a substantial risk that the baby might be born with serious physical or mental abnormalities. The number of such terminations varies markedly between different regions in the country with parts of London having the highest rate, six times that of Liverpool (6.5 per thousand women aged 15 to 49 years). Where the highest rates of termination in the National Health Service exist, up to 40 per cent of the terminations have been done privately. A high proportion of young women, pregnant for the first time, are terminated in private nursing homes. Widespread knowledge and use of contraception and sterilization are the only ways to keep the demand for therapeutic termination within manageable limits.

REFERENCES

1. Aitken-Swan, J.: Therapeutic abortion in north-east Scotland. Brit. Med. J. 2:167, 1969.
2. Baird, D.: Fertility control. Brit. J. Hosp. Med. 2:597, 1969.
3. Clark, M., Forstner, I., Pond, D. A., and Tredgold R. F.: Sequels of unwanted pregnancy. Lancet 2:501, 1968.
4. Diggory, P., Peel, J., and Potts, M.: Preliminary assessment of the 1967 Abortion Act in practice. Lancet 1:287-291, 1970.
5. Godber, G.: Safety of mother and child. Lancet 2:312, 1969.
6. Goodhart, C. B.: Estimation of illegal abortions. J. Biosoc. Sci. 1:235, 1969.
7. Huldt, L.: Outcome of pregnancy when legal abortion is readily available. Lancet 1:467, 1968.
8. Pond, D. A.: No questions asked . . .? Lancet 1:611, 1967.
9. Registrar,General: Quarterly Return for England and Wales. H. M. S. O. London, 4th Quarter 1968.
10. The Abortion Act, 1967; findings of an inquiry into the first years' working of the Act, conducted by the Royal College of Obstetricians and Gaenecologists. Brit. Med. J. 2:529, 1970.

Age, Marriage, Personality, and Distress: A Study of Personality Factors in Women Referred for Therapeutic Abortion

By Peter C. Olley, M.B., Ch.B., B.Sc., Dip. Psych. (Ed.)

D URING THE LAST THREE YEARS, the departments of Obstetrics, Mental Health, and Sociology of the University of Aberdeen have been cooperating to investigate many aspects of therapeutic abortion in Aberdeen, Scotland. Aberdeen, because of its well organized obstetric and psychiatric services, its comparatively static population and, over the last 20 years, its relatively liberal attitude to therapeutic abortion is a particularly suitable area for a comprehensive study.

Three hundred and seventy Aberdeen women, referred for consideration of pregnancy termination, were given a series of standardized psychological questionnaires to assess mental state at referral, and personality characteristics. This was the first stage of a project designed to evaluate long-term social and psychological effects of termination or continuation of an "unwanted" pregnancy.

The cohort composition (Table 1) was found to comprise 92 per cent of all Aberdeen women referred for termination to the city hospital services during the period of July 1967 to August 1968. Medical, social, and psychiatric indications were all included in the group, which was tested prior to interviews by the decision-making obstetricians and psychiatrists and following interviews by medical sociologists. Information about the social and medical background, current life situation, and the circumstances leading to the pregnancy was available for each patient. The results of follow-up interviews and testing, eighteen months after referral, are to be reported at a later date as part of an interdepartmental monograph on abortion. This paper concentrates on the results of the initial personality testing.

Three hundred and sixty-eight women completed Cattell's 16 Personality Factor Test (16 P.F.) Form C. Adult personality is described in terms of 16 essentially independent bipolar factors.[1,3,4] Each factor has a high scoring pole and a low scoring pole, representing a high degree and a low degree of the personality trait. The majority of normal populations have intermediate scores. The factors are identified by letters and brief descriptions of their personality characteristics applied to each opposing pole. It was considered that this short test, despite several inherent limitations, could give useful clues about group personality traits in the test situation.

Scoring is on a standardized ten-point scale in units called stens, calibrated against reference populations with arithmetic means of 5.5 stens and a standard deviation of two stens for each factor. Tables of norms are available for vari-

Based on a paper read to the Annual British Medical Association Scientific Meeting in Aberdeen, July 9, 1969.

Table 1.–Cohort Composition by Age, Marital and Pregnancy Status

Age in Years	Under 15	15–19	20–24	25–29	30–34	35–39	40–44	45+	Total No.	Per cent	Mean	S.D.
Number of married with legitimate pregnancy	0	3	25	51	41	33	16	1	170	45.9	31.3	6.4
Number of married with illegitimate pregnancy	0	0	6	16	7	5	3	0	37	10	30.2	5.8
Number of single	1	72	74	9	3	4	0	0	163	44.1	21.1	4.3
Total	1	75	105	76	51	42	19	1	370	100	82.6	16.5

Table 2.—Personality Factors in the 16 P.F.

Low Score (−)	Factor	High Score (+)
Reserved	A	Outgoing
Less Intelligent	B	More Intelligent
Emotional	C	Stable
Submissive	E	Dominant
Sober	F	Enthusiastic
Expedient	G	Conscientious
Shy	H	Venturesome
Tough-minded	I	Tender-minded
Trusting	L	Suspicious
Practical	M	Imaginative
Forthright	N	Shrewd
Placid	O	Apprehensive
Conservative	Q_1	Experimenting
Group-tied	Q_2	Self-sufficient
Uncontrolled	Q_3	Controlled
Relaxed	Q_4	Tense

ous general populations and patterns of scores have also been published for special populations, e.g., psychiatric patients, certain occupational groups, aggressive criminals, etc. Scores on some factors are known to vary normally with age in definite ways. Cattell's general population of non-student women was taken as the standard population.[3] Group means and standard deviations in stens were calculated on each factor for women differing on such variables as marital status, legitimacy of pregnancy, age, social class, and referral to a psychiatrist. Comparisons were made with general populations and between the groups of referred women. The significance of differences between group means was assessed by two-tailed t-tests.

RESULTS

Comparison With the General Population of Women

Ever-married women comprised married women living with their husbands, divorcees, widows, and those separated from their husbands. As can be seen from Table 4, those with legitimate pregnancies differed significantly on eight factors from the general population of nonstudent women, namely they were more *tense, apprehensive, sober, tenderminded, emotional, shy, reserved,* and *uncontrolled.* The first six of these characteristics include six of Cattell's eight "neuroticism" factors, including the five most highly loaded components.[4] The scores of married women with illegitimate pregnancies resembled those with legitimate pregnancies except that Factor 0 (*placid-apprehensive*) did not differ significantly from the general population. In addition they were less *practical, submissive,* and *trusting* than the general population. The single women scored abnormally on fifteen factors, including the neuroticism pattern, *trusting-suspicious* being the only exception.

These results suggest that all three groups are abnormal populations having a neurotic tendency in common as well as other distinguishing qualities.

Table 3.–16 P.F. Means and Standard Deviations for Marital and Pregnancy Status Groups (sten units)

		A	B	C	E	F	G	H	I	L	M	N	O	Q₁	Q₂	Q₃	Q₄
Single women N=163	Mean	5.1	6.2	4.6	6.2	4.7	4.5	4.0	6.4	5.7	6.1	6.0	6.0	6.0	4.7	3.7	7.3
	S.D.	2.3	1.5	2.1	2.4	2.0	2.3	2.2	2.1	1.9	2.1	1.9	2.1	2.2	2.0	1.8	1.9
	t_{12}	0.99	4.41	0.42	2.21	2.44	3.95	2.31	0.13	0.69	4.09	1.77	2.35	1.10	3.75	3.34	0.64
	p_{12}	N.S.	<0.001	N.S.	<0.05	<0.05	<0.001	<0.05	N.S.	N.S.	<0.01	N.S.	<0.05	N.S.	<0.001	<0.001	N.S.
Ever-married (legitimate pregnancy) N=169	Mean	4.9	5.4	4.5	5.6	4.1	5.5	4.6	6.4	5.6	5.2	5.7	6.5	5.8	5.5	4.3	7.2
	S.D.	2.3	1.7	2.1	2.4	1.9	2.1	2.3	2.0	1.9	1.9	1.9	2.1	2.1	1.9	1.9	2.1
	t_{23}	0.65	0.40	0.19	1.58	0.01	0.25	1.42	0.36	2.84	2.95	1.04	1.28	0.10	0.88	0.75	0.09
	p_{23}	N.S.	N.S.	N.S.	N.S.	N.S.	N.S.	N.S.	N.S.	<0.01	<0.01	N.S.	N.S.	N.S.	N.S.	N.S.	N.S.
Ever-married (illegitimate pregnancy) N=36	Mean	4.6	5.3	4.4	6.3	4.1	5.6	4.0	6.5	6.6	6.3	6.0	6.0	5.7	5.2	4.1	7.2
	S.D.	2.3	1.3	2.0	2.2	2.1	2.6	2.2	1.6	1.6	2.4	1.7	2.1	2.0	1.3	1.9	2.1
	t_{13}	1.22	3.24	0.44	0.27	1.39	2.4	0.05	0.41	2.4	0.48	0.03	0.1	0.74	1.47	1.24	0.49
	p_{13}	N.S.	<0.01	N.S.	N.S.	N.S.	<0.05	N.S.	N.S.	<0.05	N.S.	N.S.	N.S.	N.S.	N.S.	N.S.	N.S.

t_{12}: single v. legitimate

t_{23}: ever-married legitimate v. ever-married illegitimate

t_{13}: single v. ever-married illegitimate

Table 4.—Significant 16 P.F. Factors Compared with Cattell's General Population

16 P.F.		A	B	C	E	F	G	H	I	L	M	N	O	Q_1	Q_2	Q_3	Q_4	n
Single women	t:	2.01	3.89	4.71	3.37	4.38	5.17	7.90	4.66	1.29	3.42	2.95	2.61	2.71	4.46	10.16	10.06	
		A(−)*	B(+)	C(−)	E(+)	F(−)	G(−)	H(−)	I(+)	N.S.	M(+)	N(+)†	O(+)†	Q_1†(+)	Q_2(−)	Q_3(−)	Q_4(+)	163
Ever-married (legitimate pregnancy)	t:	3.37	0.60	5.31	0.38	7.54	0.24	4.94	4.95	0.51	1.40	0.94	5.54	1.40	0.05	6.46	9.16	
		A(−)	N.S.	C(−)	N.S.	F(−)	N.S.	H(−)	I(+)	N.S.	N.S.	N.S.	O(+)	N.S.	N.S.	Q_3(−)	Q_4(+)	169
Ever-married (illegitimate pregnancy)	t:	2.60	0.65	3.03	2.21	3.89	0.16	4.35	3.00	3.08	2.35	1.53	1.51	0.64	0.90	4.08	4.78	
		A(−)*	N.S.	C(−)†	E(+)*	F(−)	N.S.	H(−)	I(+)†	M(+)†	M(+)*	N.S.	N.S.	N.S.	N.S.	Q_3(−)	Q_4(+)	36

* = P < .05
N.S. = Not Significant
† = P < .01
Letter without asterisk = P < .001
(General population of women N = 416; for each factor Mean = 5.5 sten; S.D. = 2 sten)

Table 5.—16 P.F. Profiles for Sub-groups of Single Women (Sten Units)

		A	B	C	E	F	G	H	I	L	M	N	O	Q_1	Q_2	Q_3	Q_4
Singe women with previous pregnancy N = 31	Mean	4.8	6.0	4.9	6.5	4.3	4.8	3.9	6.2	5.9	6.4	6.5	6.3	5.7	4.7	3.3	7.4
	S.D.	2.1	1.3	1.8	2.2	2.1	2.3	2.2	1.8	1.8	2.3	1.7	1.9	2.4	2.0	1.7	1.9
Single women with lack of contraception N = 122	Mean	5.1	6.1	4.6	6.1	4.6	4.5	3.9	6.4	5.8	6.0	6.0	6.0	5.8	4.9	3.6	7.3
	S.D.	2.2	1.6	2.2	2.4	2.1	2.3	2.2	2.0	1.8	1.9	2.2	2.2	2.2	2.0	1.8	2.0

Comparison Between Groups

Single women were significantly more *imaginative, expedient, uncontrolled, assertive, intelligent, group-tied, shy, placid,* and *enthusiastic* than the married women with legitimate pregnancies. The first four factors, and particularly *imaginative* and *expedient,* figure prominently in the personality profiles of car drivers subject to repeated accidents.[1,4] This cluster may perhaps be termed "accident proneness."

Married women with illegitimate pregnancies were more *imaginative* and more abnormally *suspicious* than the married women with legitimate pregnancies. Their group means deviated notably more from the general population on *uncontrolled, dominant,* and *shy* but less on *apprehensiveness* than the legitimate group, but these differences did not reach statistical significance.

Single Women with Previous Pregnancy

Since personality traits associated with illegitimacy are likely to be more extreme in single women who have had more than one pregnancy than in women with a first illegitimate pregnancy, the group of single girls were compared in this way. Single girls with repeated pregnancies deviated more from the general population of women on *imaginative, uncontrolled,* and *dominant* characteristics than those of single women as a whole, but the differences were not statistically significant. *Expediency* was less prominent as was *intelligence,* but again to an insignificant degree.

Lack of Contraception

The 122 single women who apparently made no attempt at contraception, either themselves or via their partner, did not differ significantly from the total women's group on any of the sixteen factors—including *intelligence* (Table 5).

Among the single women applying for termination, repeated risk-taking and repeated illegitimate pregnancy was not clearly associated with inferior intellectual ability. This sample, however, may not be typical of unmarried pregnant women, and the selection process may have already occurred whereby only the more intelligent were referred.

Referral for Psychiatric Opinion

There was no difference in personality profile between 62 single girls referred for psychiatric opinion and the total group of single women on any of the sixteen factors (Table 6).

By contrast, 46 ever-married women referred for psychiatric opinion differed significantly on a number of factors from the whole group of ever-married women. They were significantly more *reserved, emotionally unstable,* and *tense.* There was also a tendency for them to be more *shy, imaginative,* and *uncontrolled,* but these differences did not reach statistical significance. Thus, this group seems to be psychologically more vulnerable than the rest of the ever-married women. On the other hand, basic personality characteristics do not appear to determine the selection of single girls for psychiatric

Table 6.–16 P.F. Profiles for women referred for Psychiatric Opinion

		A	B	C	E	F	G	H	I	L	M	N	O	Q_1	Q_2	Q_3	Q_4
Single women* N = 163 (sten units)	Mean	5.1	6.2	4.6	6.2	4.7	4.5	4.0	6.4	5.7	6.1	6.0	6.0	6.0	4.7	3.7	7.3
	S.D.	2.3	1.5	2.1	2.4	2.0	2.3	2.2	2.1	1.9	2.1	1.9	2.1	2.2	2.0	1.8	1.9
Psychiatric referrals of single women N = 62 (sten units)	Mean	4.7	6.1	4.4	5.9	4.5	4.7	3.8	6.0	5.7	6.5	6.1	6.1	6.0	4.7	3.4	7.7
	S.D.	2.4	1.7	2.2	2.2	1.9	2.1	2.0	2.0	1.9	2.2	1.7	2.3	2.1	2.0	1.9	1.8
Ever-married women N = 205	Mean	4.8	5.4	4.5	5.7	4.1	5.5	4.5	6.4	5.8	5.4	5.7	6.4	5.8	5.4	4.3	7.2
	S.D.	2.3	1.6	2.1	2.4	1.9	2.2	2.3	1.9	1.9	2.0	1.9	2.1	2.1	1.8	1.9	2.1
Psychiatric referrals of ever-married women N = 46	Mean	4.1	5.0	3.8	6.1	3.7	6.0	3.8	6.2	5.6	6.1	5.6	6.6	5.7	5.5	3.7	8.0
	S.D.	1.9	1.8	1.9	2.5	2.0	2.0	2.0	1.8	1.8	1.9	2.0	2.5	2.1	2.0	1.9	2.0
	$p34$	<.05	N.S.	<.05	N.S.	N.S.	N.S.	N.S.	N.S.	N.S.	N.S.	N.S.	N.S.	N.S.	N.S.	N.S.	<.05

*P_{12} N.S. for all factors

Table 7.—Comparison of Referred Student Group with Student Nurse Group

		A	B	C	E	F	G	H	I	L	M	N	O	Q₁	Q₂	Q₃	Q₄
Referred "students" (sten units) N = 62	Mean	5.0	7.0	4.6	6.0	4.8	3.7	4.1	6.7	5.7	6.3	6.0	5.3	6.6	4.4	3.4	7.3
	S.D.	2.4	1.4	2.1	2.5	2.0	2.3	2.2	2.1	2.0	2.2	1.8	1.9	2.1	2.0	1.7	2.1
Nursing students (sten units) N = 319	Mean	4.8	7.4	5.5	5.9	5.2	4.3	4.0	4.8	5.6	5.1	5.8	5.1	5.5	4.5	3.8	5.7
	S.D.	2.4	2.0	2.0	2.3	2.5	2.0	2.1	2.2	2.2	1.7	2.3	2.3	2.3	1.9	2.0	2.4
	p12	N.S.	N.S.	<.01	N.S.	N.S.	<.05	N.S.	<.001	N.S.	<.001	N.S.	N.S.	<.001	N.S.	N.S.	<.001

opinion, suggesting that nonpsychiatric factors, e.g., perception of the social situation by the obstetrician may be most important.

Comparison of Single Girls with Nursing Students

Since certain factors, notably *shy-venturesome, sober-enthusiastic, uncontrolled-controlled, placid-apprehensive,* and *relaxed-tense* tend to show normal age trends, an attempt was made to control for this factor. A subgroup of 62 of the single women with illegitimate pregnancies who were students were compared with a group of 319 Aberdeen nursing students who, although not perfectly matched, served as age controls. The scores of the student subgroup were significantly different from the general population on twelve factors but compared with their peer group of nursing students, they are different only on six—more *emotional, expedient, tender-minded, imaginative, experimenting,* and *tense*. This suggests that at least part of the obtained test differences between single girls and other pregnancy groups may be due to age and social class differences.

DISCUSSION

Analysis of the pattern of results suggests that there are two quite different processes involved: first, personality characteristics related to referral for abortion as opposed to a different solution and second, personality characteristics related to illegitimate versus legitimate pregnancy. All three groups of women who sought therapeutic abortion differed from the general population in several characteristics and suggest a certain personality pattern. Such women are: more *reserved* and *aloof* as opposed to *outgoing;* more *emotionally unstable* and easily upset with a low ego strength; more *sober* as opposed to enthusiastic; more *shy* and *timid,* over-reacting to threatening situations, (a trait which also involves inferiority feelings and difficulty in communicating with others); more *tender-minded* as opposed to *tough-minded,* more *uncontrolled,* impulsive, without clear identity and lacking in self-respect; and more *tense* and excitable with a tendency toward irrational worry, irritability, anxiety, and turmoil.

In contrast to the rather "neurotic" personality patterns associated with women seeking therapeutic abortion, the legitimacy versus illegitimacy of pregnancy variable seems to reflect quite a different pattern. Women with illegitimate pregnancies tend to show characteristics which have been described as accident prone. Marked differences between married and single girls are evident however. Ever-married women with illegitimate pregnancies, as compared to those with legitimate pregnancies, were more *imaginative,* absent-minded, and unconventional. This factor pole is sometimes described as "bohemian." Perceptions of the world and of other people tend to be distorted to conform with an intense inner life of fantasy. A person with this trait may become so self-absorbed that practical matters are neglected. They also showed more *abnormal suspiciousness* involving jealousy, hostility, and social insecurity.

Single girls with illegitimate pregnancies similarly differed from married women with legitimate pregnancies in the *imaginative-practical dimension* but not on the *suspicious-trusting* dimension. They were also significantly more *expedient*, undependable, changeable as opposed to *conscientious* and perservering, tending to ignore social rules and feeling few obligations toward others (a trait often found in psychopathic individuals); more *uncontrolled*, impulsive, without clear identity, and lacking in self-respect; more assertive. *dominant*, and attention-getting as opposed to humble and *submissive;* and more *intelligent*. This factor is only a rough measure of intelligence and it indicates the degree of academic capacity and sophistication. A higher score on the single women's group was to be expected because of the large portion of students. This group was also more *group-dependent* and imitative as opposed to *self-sufficient* and resourceful and more *shy* and timid, over-reacting to threatening situations. This trait also involves inferiority feelings and difficulty in communicating with others. Women with legitimate pregnancies were more *apprehensive*, insecure, and guilt-prone. This factor is among the most important ones in neuroticism. Cattell associates this trait with feelings of anxiety, depression, and a tendency to suffer internal conflict rather than act out a problem; these women were more *sober* and serious as opposed to enthusiastic and happy-go-lucky, which seems to be related to the punishment of past experience. Scores tend to decrease with age and reflect an increase in the load of worry and responsibility.

The conclusions drawn from this preliminary analysis must, of necessity, be tentative.

SUMMARY

At Aberdeen characteristics of 370 women were measured by Cattell's Sixteen Personality Factor Test (16 P.F.). The personality pattern of women who sought abortion was found to be more "neurotic" than the general population. Women with illegitimate pregnancies showed personality characteristics similar to persons described as accident prone.

REFERENCES

1. Cattell, R. B.: Personality and Motivation Structure and Measurement. New York, World Book Co., 1957.

2. —, and Eber, H. W.: Handbook for the 16 Personality Factor Questionnaire Forms A, B, and C. Champaign, Ill., I.P.A.T., 1957.

3. —: Handbook Supplement for Form C of the 16 Personality Factor Questionnaire (ed. 2), Champaign, Ill., I.P.A.T., 1962.

4. —, and Scheier, I. T.: The Meaning and Measurement of Neuroticism and Anxiety. New York, Ronald Press, 1961.

5. Cordiner, C.: Personal communication. 1970.

6. Suhr, V. W.: The Cattell 16 P. F. as a prognosticater of accident susceptibility. Proc. Iowa Acad. Sci., 60:553-561, 1953.

Abortion or No? What Decides?
An Inquiry by Questionnaire into the Attitudes of Gynecologists and Psychiatrists in Aberdeen

By C. McCance, M.A. M.B., M.R.C.P.,
and P. F. McCance, M.R.C.S., L.R.C.P., M.B., B.S.

THE ABORTION ACT (1967) provides that two medical practitioners acting in good faith can recommend an abortion on the following grounds: (1) the continuance of the pregnancy would involve risk to the life of the pregnant woman greater than if the pregnancy were terminated; (2) the continuance of the pregnancy would involve risk of injury to the physical or mental health of the pregnant woman greater than if the pregnancy were terminated; (3) the continuance of the pregnancy would involve risk of injury to the physical or mental health of the existing child(ren) of the family of the pregnant woman greater than if the pregnancy were terminated; (4) there is a substantial risk that if the child were born it would suffer from such physical or mental abnormalities as to be seriously handicapped.

It will be appreciated that society, through this Act, has placed a heavy burden of decision upon doctors, in which the borderline between social, psychological and medical repercussions is seldom clear cut. This is a decision which may be excruciating, because no sound data exist from which to estimate its results in terms of statistical probability, and because a conflict of ethical and moral considerations may exist.

Long-established tradition has directed medical endeavor primarily toward the palliation or cure of disease and so, indirectly to the improving and prolonging of life in the individual. In the field of gynecology, this has come to include also the facilitation of conception. In this role, the doctor's activities are obviously in his patient's best interests and he has very clear ethical codes to guide his decisions and to satisfy his conscience. In the case of a pregnant woman the difficulty immediately arises that there are two potential patients and if the mother is seeking an abortion, the interests of the two are opposed.

The doctor's sense of loyalty to his individual patient is not always quite so easily satisfied in the field of preventive medicine and public health, although it is in this area (rather than in the realms of curative medicine) that perhaps the greater "payoff" has come in terms of human well-being in the twentieth century. The benefits, however, are less tangible, less obvious, and tend to be unrecognized by a large section of the community.

The preventive aspects of psychological morbidity are as yet largely in the realms of speculation and the possibilities would probably be appreciated by an even smaller minority; yet, termination of pregnancy can be recommended

---

Modified from a paper presented at the Annual Scientific Meeting of the British Medical Association in Aberdeen, July 1969.

in the interests of the future mental health of the pregnant woman. It can also be recommended in the interests of other members of the family. In society's wish to liberalize abortion it is probable, though not explicit, that there is an even wider concern about what the rest of society stands to lose by embracing babies whose mothers did not want to have them. Rejected children, born out of wedlock, are a charge on society, are more likely to be unhappy, to become delinquent or neurotic. And in the background is the ominous threat of world over-population which poses such a fundamental threat to mankind.

The dispute in each case where the induction of abortion is considered is basically a three-sided affair, where the interests of pregnant woman, fetus, and society may well be in conflict. All are playing for high stakes, maybe for life and death. No wonder passions run high.

How do doctors behave in this complex situation? Do they espouse the cause of the fetus, the pregnant woman or the society, of which they are willy-nilly a member? What are their attitudes and opinions? This study scratches the surface of these problems by attempting to analyze the decisions made by a group of gynecologists and a group of psychiatrists in relation to the problems which each case presented.

MATERIALS AND METHODS

All gynecologists and psychiatrists in Aberdeen were asked to complete a questionnaire following their initial examination of each pregnant woman who sought an abortion, over the period from June 1, 1967 to July 1, 1968.

The main focuses of interest in this clinical encounter were the information obtained, the attitudes displayed, and the opinions formed. Thus, the questionnaire was devised to obtain the specialists' opinions about the patient, her physical, mental and social function, past and present; attitudes toward the present situation of the patient, her next of kin and her family doctor; the bearing of certain social factors upon the patient's health in the event of a continued pregnancy, and the effect of continued pregnancy upon her existing children; the prospects for the future child, and finally, about his own attitude toward the patient and toward his decision (see Appendix).

During this 13-month period 373 patients went to the gynecologists to seek abortion, and 283 questionnaires were completed—thus 90 were not obtained. In seven cases they were intentionally omitted, the patients being colleagues, colleagues' wives, or daughters. It has been possible to compare certain information about the group of patients whose questionnaires were not documented, with those who were. With regard to age, marital status and the decision whether or not to terminate, there was no significant difference between the two groups. No reliable data were available about social class. The six gynecologists, who saw over 30 cases each, omitted to complete a questionnaire for 16-33 per cent of their cases. This difference is not statistically significant. The inference is that all were equally cooperative and that no one person was selecting an appreciable number of cases for omission. The evidence is consistent with the hypothesis that the omissions were largely accidental and that the 283 questionnaires obtained are representative of the whole group.

During the same period, 116 patients attended the psychiatric department because an abortion was contemplated, but one consultant declined to take any part in the research. He saw 11 cases and these are excluded. Of the remaining 105, 93 were documented and 12 were missed (11.5%).

In all, there were 376 documented consultations with 322 individuals. Two hundred and thirty-one had only a gynecological opinion, and 39 had only a psychiatric opinion. Forty-nine had one of each and one patient had two psychiatric interviews. Two patients had three opinions each, two psychiatric and one gynecological and vice versa.

For the first nine months, the cases referred to the gynecologists were, where possible, seen by the specialist to whom the general practitioner referred them. In the last four months, owing to increasing demands each patient was allocated at random to a consultant.

Cases referred to the psychiatric department were not, by convention, addressed to an individual specialist and were allocated to the first available outpatient clinic.

There is obviously some possibility of bias in the allocation of patients to the gynecologists in the first nine months, but less likelihood thereafter, or with the allocation to psychiatrists. The groups of patients seen by individual gynecologists and psychiatrists were compared for age structure and marital status and did not differ significantly.

It should be appreciated that the patients seen by psychiatrists are by selection a different group from those seen by gynecologists, although the two groups overlap. It is therefore unwarranted to compare the factors which appear to move gynecologists with those which influence psychiatrists, except in the group of patients which have been seen by both.

RESULTS

Analysis of Abortion Decision in Relationship to Other Factors

Patients' Ages. Table 1A shows the age groups of patients seen by gynecologists, by abortion decision. Abortion was advised in a smaller proportion of patients under 20 than in patients 20-29 or 30 and over. Table 1B shows age groups of patients seen by psychiatrists, by abortion decision. Here the same trend is discernible but because of the small numbers in the under-20 group, there is no statistical significance.

Patients' Marital Statuses. In the same way as show in Tables 1A and B, the marital status was tabulated against the abortion decision for the group seen by gynecologists and the group seen by psychiatrists. No significant dif-

Table 1.—Relationship of Patient's Age Group with Specialist's Decision

A

Gynecologists	Yes	No	Uncertain	Totals
Under 20	20	33	3	56
20–29	75	42	12	129
30 and over	58	27	10	95
Totals	153	102	25	280*

$$x^2_4 = 15.7516$$

$$p = < .01$$

B

Psychiatrists	Yes	No	Totals
Under 20	5	5	10
20–29	38	11	49
30 and over	25	6	31
Totals	68	22	90

$$x^2_2 = 4.0765$$

$$p = .2$$

*Three cases have been omitted. No decision was made because the patient changed her mind.

Table 2.—Relationship of Patient's Apparent Certainty of Wanting an Abortion to Specialist's Decision

A

Gynecologists' decision to recommend abortion	Yes	No	Undecided
Patient sure she wants abortion	135	59	21
Patient uncertain	11	37	4
Not assessed	7	6	0

2d.f. (combining patients uncertain with those not assessed) 32.5146 p<.001

B

Psychiatrist's decision to recommend abortion	Yes	No	Undecided
Patient sure she wants abortion	67	12	0
Patient uncertain	1	10	0

Fisher p<.0001

ference was found in either group. The probabilities were 0.5 and 0.7 respectively. It would appear that this factor does not in itself carry much weight in deciding the issue.

Attitudes and Opinions of Clinicians. Table 2 shows that for gynecologists and psychiatrists there was a highly significant association between a patient's single-minded wish for an abortion and the specialist's recommendation to carry one out. Other relationships were analyzed in the same way. For gynecologists, the following factors had a highly significant association (P. < .001) with a decision to recommend abortion: (1) the presence of anxiety; (2) the presence of depression; (3) the specialist's opinion that stress from existing children threatened the health of the mother in the face of continued pregnancy and later an additional infant; (4) the opinion that work commitments were of paramount importance to the patient's well-being and would be disrupted by continued pregnancy; (5) the opinion, in single women, that parental lack of sympathy would threaten healthy adjustment.

The following factors for gynecologists had a significant association at the 1 per cent level: (1) a history of bad social function and adjustment; (2) a history of past psychiatric breakdown; (3) the opinion that continued pregnancy promised severe financial hardship. There was also an association at the 2 per cent level if there was thought to be an appreciable risk that the baby would be abnormal. There was an association at the 5 per cent level for the group seen by gynecologists, between liking the patient and recommendation to carry out abortion.

For the psychiatric assessments there was a highly significant association (p < .001) between the presence of anxiety and a recommendation for abortion. There was also a significant association (p < .01) between abortion and depression and a housing problem. Other factors did not show a significant association with the abortion decision although there were some trends which larger numbers might confirm.

In this group seen by psychiatrists, abortion was advised more often in patients who were disliked but the difference did not reach statistical significance ($p < .06$).

In neither the gynecological nor the psychiatric assessments did hints, statements or more blatant threats that they would commit suicide or would seek a criminal abortion have an association with an abortion recommendation; nor did the possibility that the continued pregnancy would threaten the marital relationship.

Abortion Decisions of Individual Gynecologists Compared with Other Gynecologists and of Individual Psychiatrists Compared with Other Psychiatrists

Figure 1 shows the proportions of each gynecologist's cases in which he did or did not recommend an abortion, or could not reach a decision. Doctors H to M and Doctor A have been grouped together for statistical analysis since each of them saw very few patients. With the exception of Doctors D and F, each one shows a significant difference, compared with his colleagues in the proportion of cases in which he advised abortion. Figure 2 illustrates the decisions made by psychiatrists. The number of patients seen by each of them was smaller than that seen by individual gynecologists and so only one (Doctor T) showed a statistically significant difference from his colleagues.

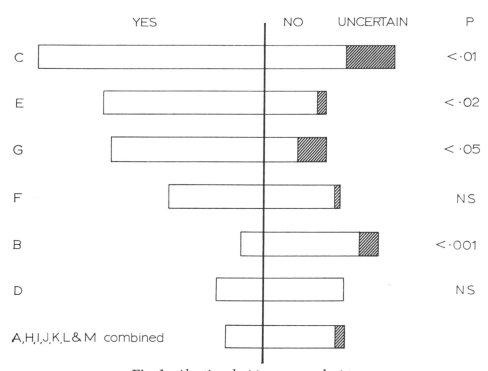

Fig. 1.—Abortion decisions: gynecologists.

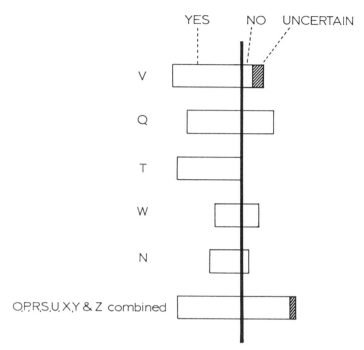

Fig. 2.—Abortion decision: psychiatrists.

Assessments and Decisions of Gynecologists Compared with Those of Psychiatrists in Group of Patients Seen by Both

There was a considerable measure of agreement between gynecologist and psychiatrist for all the following factors: depression, anxiety, threat of financial difficulty, housing difficulty, stress from the other children, history of social maladaption or psychiatric breakdown, difficulties of work commitments, feelings of the general practitioner, presence of relevant physical factors, threat of suicide or criminal abortion, patient's singlemindedness to have an abortion, the appeal of the patient as a person to the doctor and the decision about abortion (see Table 3.).

The striking difference was that the gynecologists, more often than the psychiatrists, left factors "not assessed" or were uncertain about them. This was the case for every factor except whether the patient was liked as a person. The decision about abortion is perhaps a special situation. No decision was taken by the gynecologist in 16 cases, presumably because of their referral to psychiatry.

Responses of Specialists to Research Questionnaire

There was a wide range in the extent to which the various factors suggested by the questionnaire were assessed. The presence of anxiety and depression was assessed in 99 per cent of the cases seen by psychiatrists and in 92 per cent of cases seen by gynecologists. Suicidal hints and a history of psychiatric

A   **Table 3**

	Anxiety Present	No Present Anxiety	Not Assessed	Total
Gynecologists' assessments	28	13	10	51°
Psychiatrists' assessments	29	22	1	52°

°One patient seen by two psychiatrists

B

	Patient Liked	Patient Disliked	Neutral	Not Assessed
Gynecologists	22	3	24	2
Psychiatrists	24	9	17	2

C

Abortion Recommended	Yes	No	Referred to Other Specialty without Decision
Gynecologists	20	15	16
Psychiatrists	39	12	1

breakdowns, assessments which gynecologists might have been expected to shun, were assessed by them in 82 per cent and 79 per cent of their cases, respectively. The individual "social" factors were less well assessed, by gynecologists particularly, but the greatest lack of assessment was of the husband's feelings in the married patients (only 13% assessed by gynecologists and 46% by psychiatrists), and the parents' feelings in the single girls (only 11% and 14% assessed). Another area where there was poor assessment and apparent uncertainty was concerning the feelings of the general practitioner concerned: the gynecologists had not assessed or were uncertain of his feelings in 52 per cent of cases and the psychiatrists in 36 per cent of cases.

DISCUSSION

Looking at the factors which by chance often correlate with the recommendations for abortion from either gynecologists or psychiatrists, it is interesting to see that many social factors are associated significantly with a gynecological decision to terminate pregnancy but not with the psychiatric decision. Since there was very little difference between the psychiatrists' and gynecologists' assessments in the group of patients seen by both, it seems that social problems are considered relevant by gynecologists who are prepared to make decisions on the strength of them without reference to their psychiatric colleagues. It also seems that gynecologists feel competent to proceed on their own assessment of anxiety and depression in many instances without psychiatric referral (40 and 34 cases, respectively).

It is not surprising to find the appeal of the patient's personality correlating with decisions about abortion, nor to find that doctors vary from one another in their willingness to recommend abortion. This is merely to confirm statistically what everybody knows in practice. It is perhaps a surprise to find so little divergence amongst individual psychiatrists, but in a larger series, differences might become apparent.

The last area of interest which this study seems to bring out is the large number of possibly relevant factors which have not been assessed, especially by the gynecologists. It must of course be borne in mind that the gynecological examination is brief and rushed beside the comparative leisure and calm of the psychiatric interview. Many a factor may be assessed and weighed in the gynecologist's mind without finding its way onto a time-consuming questionnaire. Nonetheless, certain factors were very regularly assessed and recorded. The implication is that they were obvious and unambiguous; the corollary is that the factors which were not well filled in were obscure and problematical. Prominent amongst these were the views of the general practitioners and of the most important relatives. It is traditional perhaps that patients hesitate to tell the doctor what they think should be done and some general practitioners perhaps feel it an impertinence to tell the hospital consultant what they think should be done. But in considering a termination of pregnancy, the unambiguous views of relatives and family doctors are vital to the proper assessment of the case. If they are not available the hospital doctor could be basing his assessment upon little else than the patient's competence as an advocate or an actress. It is perhaps relevant to recall that the patients who seemed really to want an abortion, were those in whom an abortion was more often advised.

SUMMARY

In Aberdeen a survey into the attitudes and opinions of psychiatrists and gynecologists attended by 373 women referred for therapeutic abortion was made. Questionnaires completed on 283 patients showed that anxiety, depression and social factors weigh heavily in making decisions for or against termination. Marital status, threats of suicide or resort to criminal abortion do not. The personal view of the doctor and his rapport with the patient affect his decision. Gynecologists seemed to be clearly aware of the views of the patient's doctor in less than half their cases and psychiatrists in less than two thirds, indicating a lack of communication.

APPENDIX

Check list of factors which may influence a
decision in cases for termination of pregnancy.

Patient's full name .... Date of Birth ....

Doctor completing check-list .... Date ....

1. Physical Factors: Yes   No   Not Assessed (ring appropriate)
         (If yes please state overleaf: e.g. Mitral Stenosis: Eclampsia last time).

2. Psychological Factors:
    (a) Past History of (i) Psychiatric breakdown?   Yes No N/Ass.
                   (ii) Social Maladaption?   Yes No N/Ass.
    (b) Present Mental State:
                   (i) Is there abnormal depression?   Yes No N/Ass.
                   (ii) Is there abnormal anxiety?   Yes No N/Ass.
                   (iii) Is there mental deficiency?   Yes No N/ass.
                   (iv)Is there some other morbid
                        mental state? (If yes, please
                        state overleaf)   Yes   No N/Ass.

3. Attitudes:
    (a)   (i) Does patient Exaggerate Symptoms?   Yes No N/Ass.
         (ii) Does she Threaten Suicide?   Yes No N/Ass.
         (iii) Does she Threaten Criminal Abortion?   Yes No N/Ass.
         (iv) Does she appear Unconcerned?   Yes No N/Ass.
         (v) Does she really want a termination?   Yes   No Uncertain N/Ass.
    (b) Does husband/parent/guardian (indicate which) seem to want a termination?
        (Only fill in if he/she has been seen).   Yes No Uncertain N/Ass.
    (c) Does G.P. want a termination?   Yes No Uncertain N/Ass.

4. Environmental Factors:
    Which of the following factors, if any, do you consider would affect the mental
    and/or physical well-being of the patient <u>adversely</u>, if she continued the
    pregnancy?
    (a) Financial   Yes No N/Ass.
    (b) Housing   Yes No N/Ass.
    (c) Interpersonal relationship with husband or
         putative father   Yes No N/Ass.
    (d) Stress from existing offspring   Yes No N/Ass.
    (e) Patient's work commitments or work prospects   Yes No N/Ass.
    (f) Attitudes of parents or parent substitutes   Yes No N/Ass.
    (g) Other (please state overleaf)   Yes No N/Ass.

5. Factors Concerning the Future Child:
    Is there an appreciable risk that the baby will be
    (a) Physically abnormal?   Yes No N/Ass.
    (b) Mentally defective?   Yes No N/Ass.
    (c) Liable to develop serious hereditary disease?   Yes No N/Ass.
    (d) Liable to develop serious emotional or
         personality disorder?   Yes No N/Ass.

6. Which of the above Factors were felt to be of over-riding importance?
    (e.g. 3e or 2bi and 2ai or none)

7. Did you like the patient as a person?   Yes No Neutral

8. Did you see the patient after the issue had virtually
    been decided?   Yes No

9. Did you recommend termination of pregnancy?   Yes No

The Colorado Report

By Abraham Heller, M.D., and H. G. Whittington, M.D.

T HE ENACTMENT OF A FIRST SO-CALLED MODERN LAW on therapeutic abortion by the Colorado legislature less than 3 years ago, it must be remembered, was the result of a political and legislative tour de force by a freshman member of the Colorado House of Representatives, and came about totally unexpectedly. The movement was inspired by a lay organization interested in reform of abortion laws. Legal and legislative figures, supported by a few individual physicians and some members of the clergy, led the fight. Significantly, organized medicine was not involved. The law that was enacted represented a reform of the criminal code and was patterned after the model of the American Law Institute. While most restrictive and crippling amendments were beaten down, nevertheless political necessity dictated that public policy should allow abortion only for the most serious reasons, and adopted the control mechanism which had already become entrenched in American medicine, the review board consisting of three independent physicians. In addition, the governor who signed the law served informal but clearly heard notice on the medical community that it should take care that Colorado would not become an "abortion mecca" and that abortion for any particular indication should not be "overdone."

The two major Denver newspapers, with state-wide circulation, gave strong support when the new law originally went through the legislature. The survey study under the auspices of the Colorado Psychiatric Society and the Colorado Association for Study of Abortion in the summer of 1968, compared to a similar earlier study in 1966, showed a general growth of public support for the increased availability of medical abortion.[1] Yet there is considerable controversy among professionals, as well as among the public at large. When the Denver Post recently did a series of articles sensitively and intelligently analyzing the consequences of the law, and forthrightly promoting further legal reform in the direction of abortion on demand, the letters to the editor column reflected the enormous public interest, the emotionality of the topic, and the still prevalent polarity of opinion.

Increasingly, women are raising their voices to express "the woman's view" or "women's rights" view. For many, though clearly a minority, the issue of "the rights of the fetus" is still an intensely debated issue. The allegation is that with this abortion law medicine is engaged in "killing babies."

Medicine approached its responsibilities under the new law cautiously, even timidly, and, certainly, conservatively. Only a little more than half of the accredited hospitals in the state have ever appointed an Abortion Board, such as would be required by law if the hospital were to serve therapeutic abortion cases. But more tellingly, five of these hospitals have been doing 81 per cent of all medical abortions in the state, and four of these five are in the city of Denver.

These facts reflect the uneasiness of the medical community in undertaking responsibilities under the new law. Several hospitals "went one better" than the legal requirements. They set up even more rigorous, and in effect restrictive, hospital policies than required by law. For psychiatric cases, various hospitals required recommendation by two psychiatric specialists, rather than one, as legally stipulated. At least one hospital required recommendation to the Board by three psychiatric specialists. The State Medical Society put out guidelines which militated against serving therapeutic abortion cases from outside the state, although there was no residency requirement included in the law. One important hospital would serve out-of-state cases for "medical" indications, meaning nonpsychiatric indications, but restricted its service for psychiatric cases to state residents only. The Therapeutic Abortion Committee of the State Psychiatric Society was requested by individual psychiatrists, moved by uncertainty as to their role, to set convention as to the judgment of "serious, permanent impairment of the mental health of the woman." Their wishes were opposed by those who felt that setting convention at this time would result in too conservative and restrictive application of the law. The opponents persevered and the Committee took no position, but rather left the matter open to individual clinical judgment. The composition of the Boards appointed by the hospitals also reflected the varying and sometimes uncertain attitudes. In some instances, the Boards were appointed to reflect the interested specialties, mainly obstetrics, psychiatriy, and internal medicine; in other instances the Board membership for psychiatric cases, for example, consisted only of psychiatrists.

UTILIZATION

During the first year following the passage of the law, 407 therapeutic abortions were done, for the most part, in a few hospitals, mainly in Denver.[2] Local availability of medical abortions in the rest of the state was inhibited rather than facilitated by the law.[6] This situation is now only a little improved. Almost 75 per cent of the state-wide total of therapeutic abortions are done for psychiatric indications, and inevitably reflects the concentration of psychiatrists in Denver and a few other larger communities in the state. Compared to the level prior to the passage of the law, therapeutic abortions in the first year after the passage of the law increased eightfold. By the end of 1969, the rate of therapeutic abortions had more than doubled again, and was still rising. The number at this moment is approaching 1000 per year. The increasing rate is felt to reflect the slowly growing number of hospitals which are participating, the increasing comfort of the medical profession as a whole, and of hospitals and Boards, in particular, in passing favorably upon application for abortion. At the same time public awareness has grown, and more women are disposed to utilization of medical abortion service.

Initially, there was a great deal of discomfort on all sides. A "numbers game" could be identified so that individual practitioners or hospitals, in order to defend against being identified as "abortionists," were concerned about a "respectable" rate of disapproval in order to prove that therapeutic abortion was not being made easy. More honestly, or more objectively at least, it was difficult for many physicians, conditioned by a lifetime commitment to the preservation of life, to change their lights and practice so suddenly.

In the first year following the new law, the ratio of therapeutic abortions to live births was 1.1 per cent. While therapeutic abortions have more than doubled, the number of live births have increased about 10 per cent, so that for 1969, the ratio of therapeutic abortions to live births had risen to 2.5 per cent. Even though the numbers of therapeutic abortions are running over 18 times the number done under the old law, the rate of therapeutic abortion compared to live births has scarcely moved out of the range of the national average estimated years ago,[3] and is nowhere near the rates in Scandinavian and Eastern European countries or in Japan.[2]

If, as it is widely accepted, the ratio of all induced abortions is one-fourth that of births, then we probably now have 10,000 induced abortions a year in Colorado. If so, then medical abortions are now probably 10 per cent of

FAMILY INCOME	APPROVED	NOT APPROVED
Welfare	53	39
Below $4,000	69	51
$4,000–$6,000	115	49
$6,000–$8,000	61	35
$8,000–$10,000	40	27
Over $10,000	13	13
TOTAL	351	214

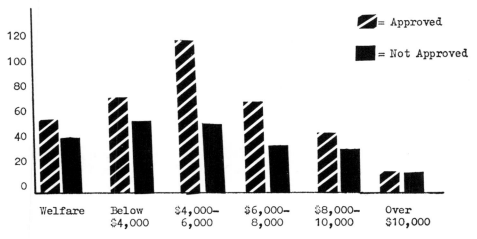

Fig. 1.—Economic class. Denver General Hospital, May 1967-February 1970.

	APPROVED	NOT APPROVED
Indian	5	0
Spanish-American	43	36
Black	66	24
Other American	237	154
TOTAL	351	214

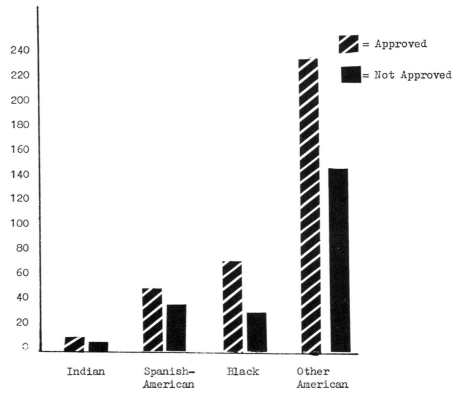

Fig. 2.—Ethnic background. Denver General Hospital, May 1967-February 1970.

all induced abortion, and are beginning for the first time to make a significant inroad in nonmedical abortion practice. Manifestly, not all of the medically aborted women would have gone the illegal route, but many would have. The likely fact is that women in this new era are more "abortion-minded," and, consequently, all induced abortions are at a higher rate. These include medical and nonmedical alike, done locally, elsewhere in this country, or abroad.

Typically, in former years, lower class women scarcely had any opportunity for therapeutic abortion. At Denver General Hospital, the average
used to be about one case per year. Now, for the first time in history numerous poor women are availing themselves of therapeutic abortion. Figure 1
indicates the breakdown according to family income. Nevertheless, even in
a hospital like Denver General which traditionally serves the poor, the utilization by this class is less than that of middle and upper class women. In
general, the poorer classes are slow to become aware and to take advantage
of the opportunities offered by new developments in medicine. In addition,
the law operates through complicated and cumbersome mechanisms which
on a de facto basis continue the traditional discrimination against the poor
and disadvantaged groups (see Fig. 2). Women who are identified with
the establishment are characteristically more determined and more able to
bend the institutions of society to their purposes.

Figures 3, 4 and 5 give the demographic characteristics of the population

	APPROVED	NOT APPROVED
Separated	28	18
Divorced	50	24
Widowed	11	3
Married	41	51
Single	221	118
TOTAL	351	214

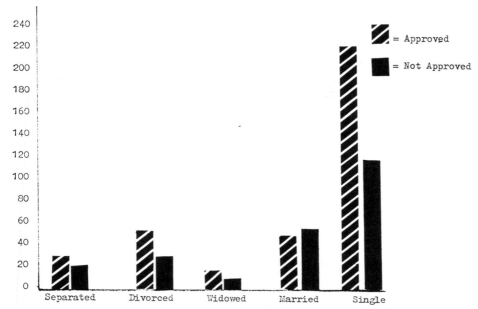

Fig. 3.—Marital status. Denver General Hospital, May 1967-February 1970.

	APPROVED	NOT APPROVED
12 - 17	97	34
18 - 21	95	73
22 - 25	64	39·
26 - 30	41	·29
31 - 35	21	23
36 - 40	19	13
41 - 42	14	3
TOTAL	351	214

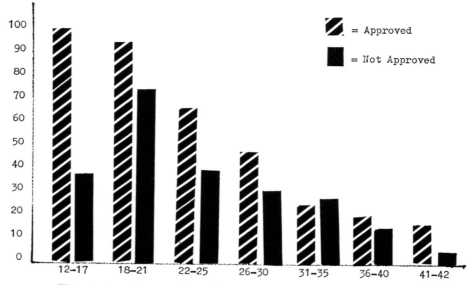

Fig. 4.—Age. Denver General Hospital, May 1967-February 1970.

served by Denver General Hospital. In contrast to previous studies in which it was brought out that the characteristic seeker of abortion was the married woman with an intact family, by far the largest group in our experience consists of single girls, half of whom are unemancipated teenagers. Prior to this era of medical practice, the case of the pregnant single girl was handled along two lines predominantly, largely determined by socioeconomic class. The middle and upper class girl often went to the home for unwed mothers where she was given considerable emotional support, and in many cases, the baby was ultimately given up for adoption. Of the girls of the ethnic minorities, predominantly of black and Spanish background in our area, and predominantly poor as well, the baby was usually delivered in the public hospitals and retained by the girl's family, usually to become part of the

	APPROVED	NOT APPROVED
None	18	16
Jewish	5	3
Catholic	91	63
Protestant	237	132
TOTAL	351	214

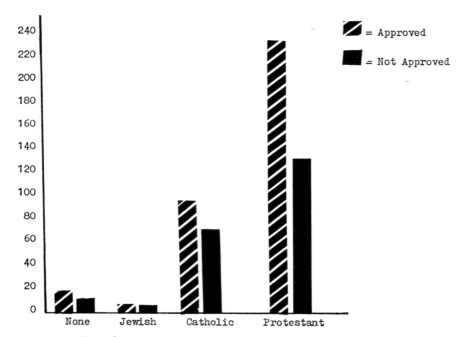

Fig. 5.—Religion. Denver General Hospital, May 1967-February 1970.

extended family of the girl's mother. The present availability of therapeutic abortion seems not to have affected the caseload activity of the homes for unwed mothers. The poorer girls still do produce "illegitimate" children which become part of extended families. Again, such therapeutic abortion practice as has developed seems not yet to have had any great impact upon these areas of life. However, within the psychiatric community, there has been the growing conviction that unwanted pregnancy for most girls through their middle teens is prima facie evidence, because of the inevitable impact upon the unfinished work of the developmental process, of serious and permanent impairment of the mental health of the girl so involved.

THE CLINICAL PROCESS

The law requires, in psychiatric cases, recommendation to the Board by one psychiatrist. Some hospitals have adopted internal rules requiring recommendation by two or more psychiatrists. The case so recommended is reported to three distinterested doctors who are appointed to the hospital Review Board, who never see the patient and consider her case in her absence. This process routinely takes about two weeks. In our opinion, this process is time consuming, costly, frustrating, demeaning to the woman, discriminatory, and inconsistent. The Board members are consciously and unconsciously subject to many subtle influences and pressures which color and give variability to their decisions. One variable is the skill with which the recommending psychiatrist advocates his case. Another is the credibility that this psychiatrist has with the Board. One hospital has taken the trouble to keep the recommending psychiatrist anonymous, but has found that method not a totally satisfactory answer to all needs. A Board composed entirely of psychiatrists will react significantly differently from one including nonpsychiatrists. Board members are troubled by such factors as personal reputations, hospital reputation, troubled conditions involving the service where the therapeutic abortions are performed, etc. They are uncomfortable in the role of having to judge their peers. Board members are also troubled by their own intrapsychic reactions, and find the assignment wearing and onerous. For all these reasons, and others, different Boards have varying rates of approval, and a given Board will go through varying phases in its own function.

One of the consequences of this time-consuming medicolegal process is that abortions, in our experience, are performed at relatively advanced gestational age, with consequent rise in complications (see Fig. 6). The suction method, which is limited to 12 weeks of gestational age, is only beginning to come into the picture. At Denver General, the vast majority of our cases are beyond 12 weeks and are done by hypertonic amniocentesis. In our hospital, as in others in the state, there has been a small but regular attendance of postabortion fever, infection, blood replacement, and occasional cases of uterine perforation. There has been no case of fatality reported in the state. Yet our Obstetrics Department informs us that with the continued use of hypertonic amniocentesis, we run the risk of an eventual, though rare, fatality.

The In-hospital Experience

Influenced by the then classical literature, we were leery in the beginning lest therapeutic abortion be attended by adverse psychological sequelae. Our investigations have been presented elsewhere and are in consonance with those of Nathan Simon and others which show that therapeutic abortion with proper screening is a psychologically safe procedure.[5,7] The law discriminates against the healthier woman in favor of the weaker, sicker one. Our studies show that therapeutic abortion patients regress under the impact of the hospital experience, and usually suffer mild, transient depression as the immediate postabortion experience. Psychotic patients are apt to become transiently more floridly psychotic under the hospital and surgical stress. All patients tolerate the procedure reasonably well, nevertheless, and

WEEKS	APPROVED	NOT APPROVED
6 – 8	25	15
9 – 11	86	47
12 – 14	120	71
15 – 17	64	41
18 – 20	52	20
21 – 30	4	20
TOTAL	351	214

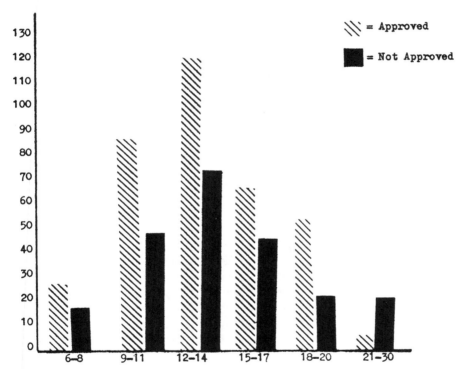

Fig. 6.—Gestational age. Denver General Hospital, May 1967-February 1970.

recoup their former equilibrium in rapid order. But the healthier the woman, the better she tolerates the entire procedure.

In most hospitals, as in Denver General, therapeutic abortion cases are handled on the obstetrical floor, sandwiched in among maternity patients. This situation is traumatic for all concerned, patient and staff. On the obstetrical floor, many of the staff do not identify positively with the woman who is being aborted on psychiatric grounds. There is apt to be a great deal

of questioning as to the medical propriety of the procedure. The cues that
the nursing staff get from their obstetrical-medical leadership often support
and maximize the ambivalence. Personal attitudes make inroads on the
professional staff's capacity to meet the legitimate needs of the patients. The
rejection, usually nonverbal but unmistakable, but occasionally even verbal
and explicit, can be devastating. This abortion procedure and this patient
are foreign bodies on the Obstetrical Service, and the resulting experience for
the patient is often less than therapeutic. Special measures have had to be
adopted at Denver General, providing in-service training for nursing and
house staff, and providing intensive ongoing liaison and consultation at the
nursing and house staff level in order to bring about a correction of the
situation.

The fate of the abortion case on the maternity floor has been further
complicated in hospitals like Denver General by the event of simply
adding a considerable new caseload onto an already overburdened and expanding service. Through previous years, therapeutic abortion practice on
the maternity floor was in the ratio of 1 : 1425 deliveries per year. The rate
of clinical burden is now on the order of 150 : 2000 deliveries. This state
of affairs is a consequence of a single hospital bearing a disproportionate load
of the therapeutic abortion practice in the state. Denver General can be said
to be performing many times its fair share of therapeutic abortion procedures.

Postabortion Care and Outcome

The Department of Obstetrics at Denver General Hospital expressed concern early in the mounting involvement with therapeutic abortions that
these patients, over 90 per cent of whom at this hospital were qualifying
on the grounds of "serious, permanent impairment of mental health," would
not receive psychiatric follow-up treatment. There was much to encourage
this concern. The patient with a history of prior psychiatric illness was the
exception rather than the rule. More often than not, the patient did not
consider herself as psychiatrically ill, and sought out the psychiatrist only
upon direction from her obstetrician, and came to the psychiatrist as part
of a necessary process in order to receive an abortion, but not because she
spontaneously saw any need for his services in other respects. In addition,
we had become deeply concerned because the process in the system was
thoroughly confusing. The woman sees four different sets of doctors at different stages of the game, each concerned with his immediate, limited area
of involvement. The patient thinks of herself as "obstetrical," but the staff of
the obstetrical service, both nursing and medical, tend to see her as "psychiatric." The prospects, under these circumstances, for continuity of care are
deplorable. In reaction, then, to the question raised by the obstetricians, we
did a cursory survey of the records and found to our amazement that, nevertheless, about two-thirds of the women did go on to receive at least some
mental health follow-up.

In the reform of the system that we have brought to bear, we now have a
full-time psychiatric nurse in liaison duty with the Obstetrical Service, working with the obstetrical staff and directly with patients. We also provide

in-service training to the obstetrical nursing staff. This element is in conjunction with a liaison psychiatrist who provides medical assistance, as well as
in-service training for the medical house staff. Even though the nurse is in
liaison and consultative capacity, in many cases she also is more than anyone
else the primary clinician. She not only establishes contact with the patients,
helps them through their in-hospital experience, but lays the groundwork
as well for postabortion mental health care in which she may continue to
have direct contact with the patients until a smooth transfer can be effected.
In this way, continuity of comprehensive care has been greatly enhanced.

We have concentrated our attention here on those patients who have qualified for and received therapeutic abortions. We are equally concerned, and
perhaps more concerned in some cases, with those whom the psychiatrist
feels are not qualified under the law, or who are turned down by the Board.
More than a few have been helped at the evaluation level to resolve their
ambivalence in favor of deciding to carry the pregnancy. They turn out to
be often grateful individuals who with some help from psychiatry generally
do well afterwards. The larger concept should be that the request for
therapeutic abortion allows a point of strategic intervention, with therapeutic abortion being one possible element of intervention. The responsibilities of comprehensive care and continuity of care are as vitally important
in regard to therapeutic abortion practice as they are to community mental
health in general.

Many people, including many obstetricians, feel that the justifiability and
effectiveness of the therapeutic abortion intervention are proved only if
the woman does not go on to have another pregnancy. This is far from true.
With mental health help, the woman may indeed become able to undertake
pregnancy constructively. The fact is that there have been a few "repeaters,"
women who came for a second round of therapeutic abortion, but they are
exceptional, and there is no need at all to be embarrassed by their doing so.
On the other hand, we believe that obstetricians are too often right in their
criticism of the psychiatrists involved, that psychiatrists tend to pay too little
formal attention to the problem of the future procreativity of the woman, and
the controls and supports which she may need in regard to them.

One of us made a modest questionnaire survey of the reactions of therapeutic abortion candidates.[8] Of 31 replies from women who have been
aborted, only two indicated that they would not make the same decision
again. Four were not sure, and 25 indicated they would make the same
decision if faced with similar circumstances. This pilot study would seem to
support the general thrust of the literature then, that, for most women, therapeutic abortion does not represent a major psychic trauma.

Our staff is involved in the follow-up of an increasing proportion of the
abortion patients. In our experience, and in the opinion of the rest of the
psychiatric community of the state as we know it, adverse reactions are
rare, and, on the whole, the women are content with having had the procedure and feel themselves benefited by it.

IMPLICATIONS FOR THE FUTURE

Medicine is again not distinguishing itself in vision and in leadership in regard to the health needs of individuals, as well as society as a whole. It is fervently to be hoped that the dismal record of organized medicine in regard to Medicare will not be repeated in regard to therapeutic abortion. The die is cast. There are simply too many people, too much pollution, too much misery, so that the survival of the human race even becomes questionable. As Dr. Alan F. Guttmacher pointed out in testimony before the Nelson Senate Committee (February 25, 1970), ". . . . one of the gravest sociomedical illnesses (is) unwanted pregnancy." Dr. Guttmacher further underlined his point, "750,000 children born each year were unwanted at the time of their conception. Undoubtedly a significant proportion led to unwanted, unloved, neglected and abandoned children."[4]

Women, just like other oppressed subgroups in society, but who are in this case a majority rather than a minority, will not remain disenfranchised for much longer. Mysogyny which has ruled much of the attitudes and laws of civilization since the beginning of time will be forced to give way. Abortion is pandemic; only a minute proportion of abortions are done under medically proper and legally sanctioned circumstances. This nonmedical practice has inflicted untold morbidity and no little mortality on the women who have felt compelled to risk it. Medicine cannot conscionably continue to condemn women into seeking relief in nonmedical abortions. Or more crassly, medicine will be forced to compete, since nonmedical abortions are constantly improving in quality.

Eight states followed Colorado in adopting some version of the American Law Institute's model law in attempting to take a liberalizing step in medical abortion practice. In addition, Maryland, in its legal reform, took a slightly different tack in transferring the matter to the medical practices code, but then proceeded to set up the same restrictions as called for by the model law. Now the state of Hawaii has passed a liberal law which puts the question of therapeutic abortion where it belongs, as a matter of medical practice, a transaction between a woman and her physician, with specialty consultation in indicated cases. Simultaneously, attacks are proceeding in the courts, and new attacks are being mounted which very likely will overturn all the laws, the old and the new which exist on the books of the various states, now excepting only Hawaii. Medicine, therefore, has to look forward to and anticipate its new responsibilities in realistic and progressive ways. Our present medical system simply cannot absorb any significant shift in the numbers of women requiring abortions.

Medicine needs to prepare and have ready in advance a system which can meet the inevitably growing numbers of abortions which women will require, and meet them efficiently, economically, under dignified circumstances and in a manner which integrates comprehensively with other aspects of health care. The system should enable the determination of the justifiability of abortion to be made much earlier in pregnancy, so that the abortion procedure becomes much more simple and more safe, physically as well as psychologically. If the bulk of the abortions could be done under 12 weeks of gestational age, most of them could be done on an outpatient basis. It may be necessary to plan upon specialty clinics to accomplish the purposes set forth here.

Finally, we have to look at the changing role of the psychiatrist in this changing world of medicine. In a complex and shifting way, psychiatry unavoidably becomes involved in all social change, especially those which affect sexual matters. It would seem that there are several distinct phases that may be identified.

a. The role of psychiatry is first to help facilitate needed social change by lending the respectability of scientific medicine to a change in social practice. This is the essence of the current role of psychiatry in providing evaluations to certify that a woman "is in danger of experiencing serious, permanent impairment to her mental health if the pregnancy is allowed to continue to term." As one of us has discussed elsewhere,[8] the scientific hope upon which this function of the psychiatrist is based may actually be chimerical. But in performing this function, the psychiatrist does contribute to the change that actually is taking place in practice.

b. As change in social practice begins, psychiatrists in medical and other social institutions are responsible for becoming therapists to the social system as such. The preceding discussion of the role of psychiatry in our setting in helping the Obstetrical Service work through the conflict in values that are necessitated by this change in medical practice would be an example of this phase.

c. Social psychiatry then has a potential role in facilitating the integration of modified social practice into the value and belief systems of individuals and organizations within society. This particularly important role is little understood and much underestimated by psychiatry as a profession. The multiple inhibitions of individuals about abortion, in addition to the institutional inhibitions and barriers, result in many women being aborted at a time when the gestation is considerably advanced, when the surgical procedures are attended with more morbidity and even some danger of mortality. Or worse, the woman does not get a medical abortion, or gets no abortion at all when she could have benefited from it. Only when the acceptability of therapeutic abortion has been fully integrated into the psychological functioning of many women in our society and the institutions that serve them will timely and safe therapeutic abortions be done, in a fully constructive experience for the woman, with a positive contribution to her health needs.

SUMMARY

Though therapeutic abortions in Colorado have increased 18-fold, the practice is still relatively limited by unreadiness and indecisiveness of organized medicine and by cumbersome and discriminatory legal mechanisms. The process is fragmented, lacks continuity of care, and subjects the woman to less than therapeutic experience. The die is cast. Medicine needs to prepare abortion services for greatly increased demands. To facilitate this, psychiatry should lend the respectability of scientific medicine and facilitate such desirable change of values and beliefs in society.

REFERENCES

1. Cobb, J. C.: Abortion in Colorado 1967-1969, changing attitudes and practices since the new law. Presented to the American Association of Planned Parenthood Physicians, San Francisco, April 10, 1969.

2. Droegmueller, W., Taylor, E. S., and Drose, V. E.: The first year of experience in Colorado with the new abortion law. Amer. J. Obstet. Gynec. 103:694-701, 1969.

3. Heffernan, R. J., and Lynch, W. A.: What is the status of therapeutic abortion in modern obstetrics? Amer. J. Obstet. Gynec. 66:335-345, 1953.

4. Guttmacher, A.: Testimony before the Gaylord Nelson Senate Committee, before the Monopoly Subcommittee of the Senate Committee on Small Business. February 25, 1970.

5. Heller, A., Tower, M., and Zahourek, R.: The phenomenology of hospital therapeutic abortion. Read at the 125th annual meeting, APA, Bal Harbour, Fla., May 1969.

6. —, and Whittington, H. G.: The Colorado story: Change in law on therapeutic abortions—Denver General Hospital experience. Amer. J. Psychiat. 125:809-816, 1968.

7. Simon, N. M., Rothman, D., and Senturia, A. G.: Psychiatric illness following therapeutic abortion. Amer. J. Psychiat. 124:59-65, 1967.

8. Whittington, H. G.: Evaluation of therapeutic abortion as an element of preventive psychiatry. Amer. J. Psychiat. 126:1224-1229, 1970.

Abortion on Request: Its Consequences for Population Trends and Public Health

By CHRISTOPHER TIETZE, M.D.

INDUCED ABORTION is statistically terra incognita in all countries where it is illegal under most circumstances. In the United States, the regulation of abortion is under the jurisdiction of the individual states. Since the laws of all states are restrictive (although in varying degrees), information on the incidence and other demographic aspects of induced abortion is grossly incomplete.

In 1957, a committee of the Arden House Conference on Abortion[2] reported that "a plausible estimate of the frequency of induced abortion in the United States could be as low as 200,000 and as high as 1,200,000 per year." The group saw "no objective basis for the selection of a particular figure between these two estimates as an approximation of the actual frequency." Over the past decade no new data have become available on which to base a more reliable estimate, let alone to assess a possible trend. Nevertheless, constant repetition has led to the wide acceptance of a round figure of 1 million induced abortions per year, corresponding to an abortion rate of 5 per 1000 population and an abortion ratio of almost 30 per 100 live births.

MORTALITY FROM ILLEGAL ABORTION

Information on deaths resulting from illegal abortion in the United States is also unsatisfactory. Estimates of 5000 to 10,000 deaths per year, still used by reputable authorities,[4] may have been valid when they were first published more than 30 years ago.[9] Today, when the total number of deaths among women of reproductive age, 15–44 years, from *all* causes is about 50,000 annually, these estimates are no longer defensible.

According to official statistics, only 189 deaths from abortion were reported for the entire United States in 1966.[16] Doubtless, most of these deaths were associated with illegal abortion, either self-induced or induced by untrained individuals. Also, additional deaths from abortion have doubtlessly been untruthfully or mistakenly reported under other diagnoses. Nevertheless, in my judgment, the true total number of deaths due to illegal abortion, recorded and hidden, cannot be much larger than twice the reported number, or about 400 per year. This estimate takes into consideration that women dying from the complications of an illegal abortion are likely to be admitted to a hospital, and that most of them are poor and have been aborted by nonmedical persons, which should minimize the need for "covering up" by the hospital staff.

Reported mortality from abortion has declined over the past third of a century from 9.1 to 0.5 per 100,000 women, 15–44 years of age.[11] This downward trend has been roughly parallel to the decline in maternal mortality, *excluding* abortion, from 388 to 24 per 100,000 live births over the same period. These parallel declines reflect primarily progress in the prevention and treatment of puerperal infection and other complications.

Mortality from abortion in the United States remains much higher among nonwhite women than among white women. The differential has increased substantially over the past three decades. In 1933, the mortality rate from abortion was twice as high for nonwhite women (15.4) as for white women (8.3); in 1966, it was six times as high (1.9 compared with 0.3). Although the mortality rate decreased for both groups, the decrease was relatively much greater for whites than for nonwhites. The higher mortality rates for nonwhite women result, at least to a considerable extent, from the poorer quality of abortionists and aftercare available to them. They are not necessarily an indication that nonwhite women resort to abortion more often than white women.

In 1933, reported deaths from abortion accounted for 24 per cent of all deaths among women of reproductive age. By 1966, this proportion had declined to 0.4 percent. In terms of mortality, then, illegal abortion is no longer a major public health problem in the United States. However, today physical survival is not our only concern and illegal abortion is still a serious threat to the quality of life, including mental health and human dignity, which cannot easily be quantified.

Mortality From Legal Abortion

To assess realistically the risk to life associated with induced abortion, competently performed in a medical setting, we must turn to the experience of countries where such operations are performed legally in large numbers and where reliable statistics can be collected by the health authorities.

Among the countries of eastern Europe, Czechoslovakia and Hungary publish the most comprehensive information on legal abortions, including mortality. In Czechoslovakia, 13 deaths occurred per 413,000 abortions during the period 1958–1962, corresponding to a rate of 3.1 deaths per 100,000 abortions. By 1963–1967, mortality had dropped to 2.5 per 100,000. Hungary reported a mortality rate of 5.6 per 100,000 legal abortions in 1957–1958; 3.3 in 1960–1963; and 1.2 in 1964–1967. The overall total amounted to 69 deaths among almost 2½ million legal abortions, corresponding to a mortality rate of 2.8 per 100,000.[10]

Mortality associated with legal abortion is much higher in northern Europe than in eastern Europe: about 40 per 100,000 in the early 1960s, based on 52,300 legal abortions with 21 deaths in Sweden and Denmark combined.[6,8] The principal reason for this difference is the fact that a substantial proportion of legal abortions in northern Europe is performed during the second trimester of pregnancy when the risk of complications is much higher than in the first trimester. In eastern Europe most legal abortions are performed during the second and third month of gestation.[15] In addition, the proportion of legal abortions performed on medical grounds is much larger in northern Europe than in eastern Europe where most women seeking abortion are presumably in good health.

ABORTION LAWS IN THE UNITED STATES

In 1963–1965, the number of therapeutic abortions, legally performed in hospitals, was approximately two per 1000 deliveries or about 8000 per year for the entire United States.[14] Because of the nationwide rubella epidemic, substantially more therapeutic abortions were done in 1964 than in either the preceding or the following year. During 1964, about 4000 pregnancies were terminated because of German measles in the first trimester of gestation, although this indication was not at that time officially recognized by any state.

Prior to 1967 the laws of most states stipulated a threat to the life of the pregnant woman as the sole legal ground on which abortion could be performed. Since 1967, ten states have enacted new laws relating to abortion. All of these new laws are based, with various modifications and restrictions, on the Model Penal Code of the American Law Institute (ALI). The code states that a "licensed physician is justified in terminating a pregnancy if he believes there is substantial risk that continuance of the pregnancy would gravely impair the physical or mental health of the mother or that the child would be born with grave physical or mental defect"[1] and also in cases of rape, including statutory rape, and incest.

Implementation of these new statutes has varied widely among states, among communities within the same state, and among hospitals within the same community. In some places the numbers of abortions performed in hospitals have increased tenfold during the first year of the new law; in others, there appears to have been little or no change. There is evidence, however, that even without legislation the old laws are now interpreted more liberally by the medical profession, and that the number of hospital abortions has increased significantly, at least in some places.[3] A rough estimate for 1969 suggests a total on the order of 25,000 therapeutic abortions for the entire country, compared with 8000 annually in 1963–1965.

Because the number of abortions likely to be performed under laws patterned after the Model Penal Code of the ALI falls far short of the estimated total of illegally induced abortions of perhaps 1 million, many individuals and organizations, including some physicians and such groups as the American Public Health Association and the Planned Parenthood Federation of America, now advocate repeal of abortion laws rather than reform. While repeal in the state legislatures may not be a realistic prospect at this time, relief may come from the courts. In the fall of 1969 a federal judge found the abortion statute of the District of Columbia unconstitutional, and several test cases were initiated in New York and elsewhere. Eventually one or more of these cases will reach the Supreme Court of the United States. While the decision of the Court cannot be predicted, it is important to evaluate the possible consequences of radical changes in the availability of induced abortion for population trends and public health in the United States. The following assessment is based partly on a priori reasoning, partly on the experience in countries where such major changes have actually occurred.

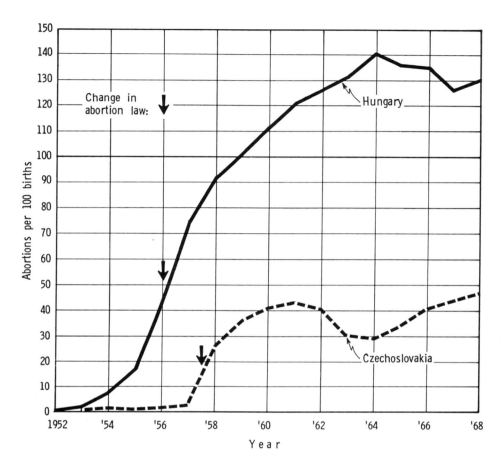

Fig. 1.—Legal abortions per 100 live births. Hungary and Czechoslovakia 1952-1968.

Changes in Abortion Laws Abroad[11,13,15]

A number of countries have abandoned their restrictive legislation and practices to permit abortion on request or on broadly interpreted social indications: the USSR in 1920 and again in 1955; Japan in 1948; and, several countries in eastern Europe during the middle 1950s. Two countries have experienced major shifts from highly permissive to substantially more restrictive legislation and practice: the USSR in 1936 and Romania in 1966.

The experience in the countries of northern Europe over the past 30 years is less relevant to our discussion because the laws in these countries are far less liberal than in eastern Europe or in Japan, and the numbers of legal abortions have been relatively small. In the United Kingdom, where a liberal abortion law came into effect in 1968, the experience has been too short for a definitive evaluation.

EFFECT ON LEGAL ABORTIONS

In all countries where the laws were changed to permit abortion on request or on broadly interpreted social indications, spectacular increases in legal abortions occurred. While reliable statistics are available for a few countries only (Fig. 1), the number of legal abortions exceeds or has exceeded the number of live births in Hungary and Romania and probably also in the USSR and in Japan. In the latter country a steady decline in the number of abortions has been reported from a peak of 1,170,000 in 1955 to 747,500 in 1967. Since many abortions in Japan are performed in doctors' offices rather than in hospitals, the completeness of reporting has been questioned by Japanese scholars.[5]

Some light on this question has been shed by the data on births and abortions in Japan for 1966. A precipitous drop in the birth rate in that year is generally attributed to the fact that 1966 was the "Year of the Fiery Horse" which occurs every 60 years, according to the traditional Chinese calendar, still widely used in Japan. Girls born in the "Year of the Fiery Horse" are believed to be very stubborn and it is difficult to find husbands for them. In this situation one would expect a rise in abortions. Instead, the reported numbers continued to decline. This would suggest that the reduction in births was achieved mainly by contraception and poses the dilemma that either the most tradition-bound segment of Japanese society practised contracepion successfully, or that the reported decline in abortions is, at least in part, a statistical artifact.

EFFECT ON ILLEGAL ABORTIONS

The effect of increased availability of legal abortion on the frequency of illegal abortion cannot be established unequivocally because the numbers of illegal abortions either before or after the legislative change are not known. Nevertheless, three generalizations are possible:

a. Moderate extension of the indications for abortion, as under the 10 new state laws based on the Model Penal Code, involves a comparatively small proportion of pregnancies and has, therefore, but little effect on the number of illegal abortions.

b. Legal abortions at the request of the pregnant woman or on broadly interpreted social indications substantially reduce the frequency of illegal and/or self-induced abortions, as evidenced by rapidly declining numbers of deaths from abortion. When Hungary and Czechoslovakia adopted liberal abortion policies in the 1950s, reported mortality from abortion declined by one-half and three-fourths, respectively, in the course of a few years. No such declines occurred over the same period in European countries with restrictive legislation.[10]

c. Illegal and/or self-induced abortions have not disappeared even in countries, such as Hungary, where abortion on request has been available for more than a decade. This stubborn survival of practices detrimental to health probably reflects dissatisfaction with the manner in which the official abortion services are organized, especially in regard to the protection of privacy.

Effect on Total Induced Abortions

Greater availability of legal abortion tends to increase the total frequency of induced abortion, which includes legal and illegal abortion, for three obvious reason: first, some pregnancies are aborted which otherwise would have been carried to term; second, these women are able to conceive again earlier than after term delivery; and third, the motivation to practice contraception is reduced. While the last effect appears to have been of some importance in a few countries of eastern Europe, there is no way to predict the response of a population accustomed to the use of modern contraceptive methods or if effective contraceptive services are provided. In at least one country (Japan), the practice of contraception is known to have expanded substantially since abortion became freely available about 20 years ago.[7]

Effect on Births

Increased availability of abortion has been followed by declines in the birth rate which, in some countries, such as the USSR in 1936 and Romania in 1966, were perceived as contrary to the national interest and led to restrictive legislation. It would be simplistic, however, to ascribe declines in birth rates entirely to changes in abortion policy. Levels and trends of birth rates are determined by broad social forces; availability of abortion merely facilitates response to these forces. If abortion had not been legalized, it is possible that declines in birth rates, achieved by more widesprad use of contraception and more frequent illegal abortion, would have been somewhat smaller. Restrictive legislation in the USSR and Romania was followed by at least a temporary reversal of the decline in the birth rate.

Effect on Mortality and Morbidity

The effect of increased availability of abortion on mortality and morbidity is the combined result of the reduced risk to life and health associated with abortions performed competently in a medical setting (as compared with those done clandestinely), and the expected increase in the total number of legal and illegal induced abortions. As long as the effect of the first factor is greater than the effect of the second, the overall trends of mortality and morbidity may be expected to decline, especially if most legal abortions are performed early in pregnancy. As stated previously, this was the experience in such countries as Czechoslovakia and Hungary following the adoption of liberal abortion policies. An opposite effect of greater availability of abortion —increased mortality and morbidity—is possible, and indeed may have occurred, in countries with a very large increase in the abortion rate, such as Romania, where abortions out-numbered births at a ratio of four to one in 1965.

Summary

It is difficult to project the consequences of radical changes in the availability of induced abortion in a population with a long tradition of contraceptive practice and comparatively easy access to highly effective methods, such as the population of the United States. One would expect that most American couples would continue to consider contraception the preferred method of birth prevention and abortion an unwelcome remedy when contraception fails. The adoption and implementation of legislation permitting abortion at the request of the pregnant woman has probable consequences for population trends and public health. Based on experience in several countries, a sharp increase in legal abortions is expected, partly at the expense of illegal abortions. The total number of induced abortions would, therefore, increase at a much slower rate than legal abortions alone. If the use of contraception were maintained at or near its present level after the legalization of abortion, the increase in the number of abortions would be moderate and the number of deaths from abortion, and of nonfatal complications as well, would be substantially reduced. The birth rate would also be lower. One would hope that this might be the outcome, but hope is no substitute for experience.

REFERENCES

1. American Law Institute: Model Penal Code: Proposed Official Draft. July 30, 1962, p. 189.

2. Calderone, M. S. (Ed.): Abortion in the United States. New York, Hoeber-Harper, 1958, p. 180.

3. Erhardt, C. L., Tietze, C., and Nelson, F. G.: Therapeutic abortions in New York City. Studies in Fam. Plan. 51:8-9, 1970.

4. Kummer, J. M. (Ed.): Abortion: Legal and Illegal. Santa Monica, Calif., J. M. Kummer, 1967, p. 21.

5. Muramatsu, M.: Effect of induced abortion on the reduction of births in Japan. Milbank Mem. Fund Quart. 38:153-166, 1960.

6. Olsen, C. E., Nielsen, H. B., Østergaard, E.: Abortus provocatus legalis: en analyse af 21,730 anmeldelser til sundhedsstyrelsen 1961-1965. Ugeskrift for Laeger. 129:1341-1351, 1967.

7. Population Problems Research Council: Summary of Ninth National Survey of Family Planning. Tokyo, Mainichi Newspapers, 1968.

8. Sweden: Medicinalstyrelsen: Allmän Hälso-och Sjukvård, 1960-66. Stockholm, 1962-1967.

9. Taussig, F. J.: Abortion: Spontaneous and Induced. St. Louis, Mosby, 1936, p. 28.

10. Tietze, C.: Abortion laws and abortion practices in Europe. In Sobrero, A. J., and McKee, C. (Eds.): Advances in Planned Parenthood V. Amsterdam, Excerpta Medica Foundation, International Congress Series 207:194-212, 1970.

11. —: Deaths from abortion in the United States, 1933-66. In Lucas, R. (Ed.): Abortion: Legal, Medical, Social, and Religious Aspects (in preparation).

12. —: The demographic significance of legal abortion in Eastern Europe. Demography 1:119-125, 1964.

13. —: Induced abortion as a method of fertility control. In Behrman, S. J., Corsa, R., and Freedman, R. (Eds.): Fertility and Family Planning. Ann Arbor, University of Michigan Press, 1969, pp. 311-337.

14. —: Therapeutic abortions in the United States. Amer. J. Obstet. Gynec. 101: 784-787, 1968.

15. —, and Lewit, S.: Abortion. Sci. Amer. 220:21-27, 1969.

16. United States: National Center for Health Statistics. Vital Statistics of the United States, 1966. Washington, D.C., 1968, Vol II, Part B, p. 124.

The Changing Practice of Abortion

By R. Bruce Sloane, M.D., and Diana F. Horvitz, B.A.

THE REVOLUTION OF VALUES about abortion, of which Stone speaks, and the rash of legislative action are changing the scene so rapidly that this book may be anachronistic before it is in print. However, the experience in New York State is likely to answer many of the questions raised in these chapters. There, after much controversy, emotional debate, and some political risk-taking, probably the most liberal and nonrestrictive abortion law in the United States was passed in 1970. This law made abortion a private matter between doctor and patient and wiped out a nineteenth-century law (1828) which allowed no abortion except to save a life. It did not stipulate a residential requirement nor where the abortion might be performed.

> ... an abortional act is justifiable when committed upon a female *with her consent* by a duly licensed physician acting (a) under a reasonable belief that such is necessary to preserve ... her life ... , or, (b) *within twenty-four weeks from the commencement of her pregnancy ...*[16]

Although it is still too soon to assess the workability of such a law, which itself remained silent on the matter of guidelines and standards, several problems are immediately apparent. There is the possibility that New York City, with more than 50 per cent of the hospital beds in New York State, may be heavily burdened with the abortion business from both residents and nonresidents of the state. The liberality of the law has made it open to both interpretation and guidelines set by several sources. Their aim is to make abortion medically sound, but these varying interpretations and guidelines create the risk of procedural delay and costs which may make abortion unavailable to the poor who often need it the most. Another consequence of the legislation has been political and religious divisiveness surrounding the morality of the law.

RESPONSE AND CONTROVERSY

Politically, legislators from Roman Catholic areas risked their careers in voting for the bill, and at least two were not returned to public office, including the Democratic Assemblyman, George Michaels, who cast the deciding vote. The governor of New York who supported the bill by signing it into law was picketed upstate by the American Society for the Protection of the Unborn. A newly formed party, the Right to Life Party symbolized by a picture of a baby in the womb, expressed its criticism of the law by seeking a place on the ballot in the New York election.

Pope Paul referred to the legalization of abortion as a "throwback to barbarianism" and likened the procedure to euthanasia and infanticide.[12] In the wake of the New York legislation, abortion has even been labelled "murder," and the state's Roman Catholic bishops called upon the governor to veto the bill. Some of these bishops have cautioned Roman Catholic physicians, nurses and medical personnel against participating in abortions.

Such reaction was to be expected and does not seem to have affected the workings of the act. Moreover, not all response to the bill has been critical, and, as part of the liberal movement, soon after the passage of the New York law, the American Medical Association amended its position on abortion, allowing (but not "requiring") doctors to perform abortions without violating medical ethics as long as they complied with applicable rules and observed good medical practice. This 1970 statement eliminated the 1871 A.M.A. ruling which committed the physician to "rid" society of the practice of abortion. The present position of the American Medical Association is open to liberal interpretation by physicians who may wish to perform abortion for social and economic reasons.

Planned Parenthood of New York City and many other public and private social agencies dealing with the unwanted pregnancy have been offering abortion counseling, information and referral service to women from all over the country, often by telephone on a 24-hour-a-day basis. Planned Parenthood publishes *Legal Abortion: A Guide for Women in the United States* which lists sources of free advice and referral in the United States and explains abortion in a simple, straightforward, almost enthusiastic manner: "Remember, if you want an abortion, have it done early!"[7] Less desirable may be the development of medical middlemen who offer women a referral service for a fee, but all these organizations are swelling the tide of applicants.

WHAT IS HAPPENING?

If numbers alone could tell the story, it could be said that New Yorkers as well as out-of-staters are getting abortions quickly, easily and in great numbers. Twenty-four hours after the law went into effect, 147 abortions were performed in 42 public, voluntary and proprietary hospitals in New York City and the upstate area.[8] This figure does not take into account those abortions performed in doctors' offices and not reported. Within 1 week the number of abortions performed in New York City municipal hospitals alone jumped to 207[9] and within 2 weeks the municipal waiting list exceeded 679.[10] At the end of 4 months of operation under the new abortion law, New York City Health Service Administration officials estimated that 50,000 abortions were performed in New York City municipal, voluntary and private hospitals along with several abortion service clinics without much strain on them and with a high degree of safety.[13] At present, physicians are required to file a death certificate for the aborted fetus. Not all doctors who had been performing abortions in their offices had been doing this, and at present there is no way to determine the total number of legal abortions performed since July 1 or to detect abortions done in doctors' offices. Abortions done outside hospitals were prohibited by the New York City Board of Health in October 1970.

An encouraging sign, health officials report, has been the decrease in waiting lists and in the backlog of abortion applicants. Most abortions in New York

City are being performed in the first 12 weeks of pregnancy, when women can be treated on an outpatient basis. Officials have set a 10-day time limit on lag between the abortion and day of initial request and have mandated that no woman be refused because of inability to pay or not be given a specific appointment. A little over a third of known hospital abortions (13,000 out of 37,000) were performed on low-income patients, and the figures reveal a high percentage of out-of-state residents.[13]

Although the complete breakdown for the 4-month figures is not available, at 2½ months of operation under the new law, approximately one-third of the known number of hospital abortion patients were nonwhite or Puerto Rican, two-thirds were less than 12-weeks pregnant, and three-quarters were between 15 and 29 years of age.[11] The Health Administration also reported that a progressively larger proportion of abortions were being performed early in the pregnancy.

New York State, and particularly New York City, will no doubt assume more than their share of the abortion business. After 3 months of legal abortion, the New York State Department of Health estimated that well over 60 per cent of all abortions in New York State had been done in New York City.[19] In one New York City hospital alone, five times as many abortions were performed as in the whole city of Buffalo. It can probably be expected that at least 50,000 nonstate residents will come to New York City annually for abortions.

A later statewide report[14] placed the actual number of *reported* abortions in New York State at 34,175 at the end of 4 months. Almost a third of these (12,607) were performed on nonstate residents; New Jersey, Massachusetts, Florida, Ohio, Illinois, Connecticut, Michigan, Indiana, Pennsylvania and Canada contributed the largest numbers of patients. It is not at all surprising that all of these states consider saving the life or health (Massachusetts) of the mother as the only justification for abortion. It is likely that New York State either will provide the example for reform in other states or will become the abortion capital of the nation. In view of this influx from out of state and the large number of illegal abortions presumed to have occurred in New York State prior to the act, how medical facilities will cope with this problem remains to be seen. Meanwhile, the preliminary findings reflect a positive picture of safe abortion for young and mostly unmarried women of various ethnic groups who are early in their pregnancy and not necessarily residents of New York State.

RESTRICTIVE GUIDELINES

The New York abortion law does not define standards and guidelines to be followed by physicians and hospitals. The New York State Department of Health, the New York City Board of Health, the State Medical Society and the Committee on Public Health of the New York Academy of Medicine have all agreed that abortion after 12 weeks should be performed on an inpatient basis only. The State Medical Society has also warned of the dangers of abortion after 12 weeks and has set 20 weeks as the limit, following which, it maintains, abortion becomes a birth process. The New York Academy of Medicine has suggested that priority for hospital abortions be given city residents or patients of city physicians and that no physician or other medical personnel be forced to participate in abortion.[3]

The New York City Board of Health prohibited abortion in doctors' offices in October, restricting the operation to hospitals, hospital-affiliated clinics or independent clinics with strictly specified staff, operating-room equipment, blood supply and laboratory equipment. Critics claimed that such restriction might eliminate a relatively cheap and expedient source of help for women who do not wish, or cannot afford, to proceed through the routine of hospital or clinic. Nevertheless, the morbidity of the precedure, although low, and at least one publicized death following treatment in a doctor's office, amply justify such limitations assuring the safety of the patient.

Gynecologists with increasing experience under the new law[15] point out that a procedure has been legalized that may require a great amount of blood, since the gravid uterus is probably the best source, second only to severing a major blood vessel, of massive hemorrhage during operation. They advise that at least two units of blood should be cross-matched and set aside for every patient and doubt whether many gynecologists would accept abortion up to the 24th week as a reasonably safe procedure. In practice, most gynecologists will not terminate a pregnancy beyond 20 weeks of gestation. Such considerations would indicate inpatient treatment in a well-equipped facility. Blue Cross and Blue Shield of New York, the state health insurance program (Medicaid) and the state employees' health insurance program have all allowed coverage for hospital abortion. This coverage is available for both single and married women, and the State Medical Society has suggested fees of $200 to $250 for inpatient care, in contrast to their recommendation of $100 to $150 for outpatient abortion.

How Safe is the Procedure?

The physical dangers incurred by the many thousands of patients now being legally aborted in New York and other states are becoming established. Even in the best of hands and with the best of facilities, abortion is not a benign procedure—but neither is childbirth. In New York State, the abortion death rate of 33 per 100,000 is slightly higher than the maternal death rate of 32 per 100,000.[14] In New York City, where the maternal death rate under hospital conditions is 10 per 100,000,[13] the figure rises to 22 per 100,000 if all eleven reported abortion-related deaths are included. (Four deaths occurred following in-hospital procedures, and seven resulted from abortion begun outside hospitals, including one in a doctor's private office.) In Britain[1] a mortality rate in the first year of the Abortion Act of 30 per 100,000 was higher than the maternal mortality rate of 24 per 100,000 which included abortions, criminal or otherwise, for all pregnancies. Notable were the two deaths from suicide, which at 7.3 per 100,000 were somewhat above the expected rate.

Unfortunately, despite the 27,331 abortions performed in Britain in the first year of the Act, it was impossible to get figures on the relative incidence of complications.[1] However, the gynecologists involved rated the following complications in order of their incidence and importance: retained products of conception, pelvic infection, puerperal pyrexia, hemorrhage, perforation of the uterus, deep venous thrombosis and embolism. Of course the risk of any complication increases markedly with the length of pregnancy, and in Britain more than one-third of the women were more than 13 weeks pregnant. In New York City,[13] fo rexample, the complications—mostly hemorrhage, infection and perforated uterus—increased from 8.2 per 1000 for women less than 12 weeks pregnant to 26.5 per 1000 after 12 weeks. Compared to results from other cities, however, the reported incidence of complications is almost unbelievably low.

Among the most important immediate physical complications in New York City are these:

1. Severe hemorrhage, which occurred in only 0.18 per cent[13] compared to 6 to 8 per cent of patients in Colorado and Aberdeen[4,5] (the latter incidence demands the transfusion services of a well-equipped inpatient facility).

2. Uterine sepsis, which occurred in only 0.24 per cent[13] compared to an incidence of from a few to 10 per cent of patients[4,5] and is seemingly more common with amniocentesis (saline replacement); usually such infections are readily responsive to antibiotic drugs.

3. Uterine perforations, which occurred in 0.24 per cent[13] compared to over 1 per cent of cases[4] in the first year's experience on Colorado where four of five patients required exploratory laporotomy, again suggesting the need for a fully equipped hospital and operating room.

Figures are not given in New York for the following complications:

4. Overt cervical lacerations, which occurred in 1 per cent of cases;[5] it is likely that in a number of other cases the cervix is damaged without the injury being suspected.

5. Thromboembolic disease, which occurred in about 1 per cent of patients[5] and is a particular complication of late cases.

It is possible that there is some underreporting of complications in New York City. This is usual in large-scale studies. It seems possible that the true incidence is closer to the Colorado and Aberdeen figures.

Although suction for early pregnancies and instillation of hypertonic saline into the amniotic sac (amniocentesis) in more advanced cases seem to be the methods of choice, and perhaps safer than earlier methods, they carry their own hazards. Fullerton[5] believes vaginal termination is more difficult than hysterotomy (transabdominal approach to the uterus) in women who have not had children. However, Kalodner[6] points to the fact that hysterotomy carries with it all the dangers and complications of a major Caesarian section, including a resultant uterine scar that may influence future pregnancies and deliveries. In addition to the immediate complications, he points to later ones such as incompetence of the cervical os—with inability to carry to term, induced secondary sterility, and menstrual irregularities. He concludes by quoting the report of the British Medical Association committee that therapeutic abortion is not a simple operation:

... mishaps will occur and they will be kept to a minimum only when operations are performed in well-equipped hospitals by skilled gynecologists who are well aware of the dangers.[17]

This warning from a widely experienced proponent of therapeutic abortion should be heeded. Such risks, however, must be set against Tietze's figures, quoted by Pohlman, of approximately three deaths per 100,000 hospital abortions in nations where physicians are experienced in abortion and where abortion is done early in pregnancy, compared to approximately 20 per 100,000 deaths in the United States from problems associated with pregnancy and birth excluding abortion.[18] Kalodner's prediction that rates in the United States are likely to be higher, both because abortion is more difficult to get and thus tends to be performed after the 12th week and because United States physicians are less experienced with the procedure than Japanese or Eastern European ones, has in fact been borne out by the results in New York State. Nevertheless, the extremely low mortality rate of abortion in New York City compared to that in Britain is most encouraging, particularly when there is little difference in the proportion of early-to-late terminations.

The Opinion of Gynecologists

Most gynecologists have been reluctant to entertain the wholesale abortion business. Such views seem to be reinforced by increased abortion practice. The report from the Royal College of Obstetricians and Gynecologists[1] on how the Abortion Act in Britain worked in the first year showed that the majority of their members thought increasing abortion would hamper both the number and quality of recruits into the specialty. If this were true, there might be serious consequences for a specialty already bedeviled by problems of recruitment. The complications of the operation and the death rate would scarcely commend its relegation at this point to lesser-trained personnel. The majority of the British gynecologists favored further restriction of the law with removal of the social clauses and were solidly against abortion on demand. They did not consider that the extramarital nature of the conception provided an acceptable indication for termination of pregnancy. They thought it was "as irrational as it was strange that a society which tolerated sexual freedom and liberal termination of pregnancy and which boasted of its concern for the rights of the individual ... should remain so intolerant to unmarried mothers and to children born out of wedlock." Nevertheless, it is unlikely that the social mores of this country or Britain will quickly change, much as the British gynecologists might desire it.

Conclusion

Our contributors emphasize that therapeutic abortion is a relatively safe procedure, both physically and mentally. At present, in both this country and Britain the physical hazards may outweigh the emotional ones.

Where the law is restrictive, the rich get abortions; the poor, especially the unmarried poor, do not. If the law is liberalized but still restrictive, the poor are still discriminated against. Doctors and hospitals, uncertain of their liabilities under the new acts, either refuse to participate or set up cumbersome tribunals and quotas that lead to delay, added cost, and added risk. Where the law is very liberal, as in Britain, its workings seem not entirely felicitous. It produces a death rate greather than carrying to term and has not reduced the incidence of illegal abortion[1]. Abortion alone, however, cannot solve the problem of unwanted pregnancies which, as our contributors point out, may be alleviated by better sexual and birth-control education. The rising tide of abortions in Britain, doubling in 1969 to 54,000 a year and, if present rates keep up, to 80,000 in 1970,[2] suggests that this is not yet happening there. The *British Medical Journal* complains that many people are unreasonable and lack foresight: "They may well be the most likely to neglect contraceptive measures and to think abortion will brighten their day as harmlessly as a shampoo."[2]

Religious beliefs and the disinclination of some obstetricians to terminate life are views that will be respected. Those who have these views should not need a law to uphold them; those who do not may not wish to have such a law. Nevertheless, the hardening inimical attitude of British gynecologists should not go unnoted. With each abortion request, they are required to make a decision involving weighing the dangers of the operation against what it may offer to health. If abortion is available on demand, the problem ceases to be a medical one except for the gynecologists' training and skills necessary for safe operative treatment and the management of complications. When abortion is available by relatively simple nonsurgical methods, as is likely in the near future, this need for expertise would be removed. Nevertheless, if there were no law concerning abortion, as some plead, it is likely that the decision, like any other medical one, would be influenced by the opinion of the physician.

Increase dabortion is likely to lower both the birthrate and eventually the morbidity surrounding birth and abortion and thus inescapably to lead to a healthier nation. In the light of present evidence, most would seek liberalization of the law that would still contain a conscience clause. It is likely that some restriction of the availability of abortion after viability of the fetus should prevail. Legalization of the procedure allows for collection of demographic facts to guide the future. Where reforms have been passed, the debate on the moral issues of abortion appears to be fading but is replaced by controversy over the complexities and shortcomings of the new laws. The possibility that nullification by the courts would leave states without laws at all is adding a new impetus that seems destined to rewrite abortion laws in every state. In view of the unsatisfactory experience with halfway measures, it is likely that many will follow the liberal lead of New York State where, although most of the sources of information to date are more journalistic than scientific, the act seems to be working well. Time alone will show how well. A betting man would probably wager in its favor.

REFERENCES

1. (The) Abortion Act (1967): Findings of an inquiry into the first year's working of the act conducted by the Royal College of Obstetricians and Gynecologists. Brit. Med. J. 2:529-535, 1970.

2. Consultants' report on abortion (editorial). Brit. Med. J. 46:491-492, 1970.

3. Committee on Public Health of the New York Academy of Medicine: Statement on implementation of the New York State abortion law. Bull. N.Y. Acad. Med. 46:674-675, 1970.

4. Droegemueller, W., Taylor, E. S., and Drose, Vera E.: The first year of experience in Colorado with the new abortion law. Amer. J. Obstet. Gynec. 103:694-702, 1969.

5. Fullerton, W. T.: Methods of abortion. J. Biosoc. Sci., forthcoming.

6. Kalodner, A. L.: Gynecologic complications of therapeutic abortion. Unpublished.

7. Langmyhr, G., and Rogers, W. C.: Legal Abortion: A Guide for Women in the United States. New York, Planned Parenthood Federation of America, 1970, p. 2.

8. New York Times, July 2, 1970, p. 1:2.

9. New York Times, July 9, 1970, p. 75:3.

10. New York Times, July 14, 1970, p. 13:1.

11. New York Times, September 17, 1970, p. 43:3.

12. New York Times, October 13, 1970, p. 2:4.

13. Report of the Health Services Administrator. New York City Department of Health, November 24, 1970.

14. Report of the New York State Department of Health to the Public Health Council. New York City, December 17, 1970.

15. Richardson, P. A., Comstock, E. F., and Kolisch, P.: Abortion and the hospital. New York State J. Med. 70:2144-2145, 1970.

16. (The) State of New York: Assembly Senate Bill 8556-A, March 23, 1970.

17. Therapeutic abortion (editorial). Brit. Med. J. 4:787, 1968.

18. Tietze, C.: Mortality with contraception and induced abortion. Studies in Family Planning 45:6-8, 1969.

19. Weisel, B. (Hospital Affairs Consultant, New York State Department of Health): Personal communication, November 9, 1970.

Index

Abortion, after rape, 87
Abortion, as criminal act, 40, 41, 54
Abortion, as complicated medical procedure, 16
Abortion, circumstances surrounding, 177-179
Abortion, ratio of live births, 153, 170
Adolescence, pregnancy in, 87-88
Age group of abortion patients, 87, 131, 144, 156
American Law Institute proposal on abortion, 24, 26, 28, 41-44, 55, 162, 167
American Medical Association, position on abortion, 173
Attitudes of poverty-level blacks on abortion, 99-107
Availability of abortion, effects of, 16-17, 44, 110-112, 117-118, 169-170

Black position on abortion, 32

California abortion laws, 32, 43, 55
Chile, abortion in, 111, 120
Colorado, abortion in, 7, 8, 151-164
Complications from abortion, 10-11, 158, 174-177
Concern with health of mother, 39-40, 43, 88
Concern with life of fetus, 38-39
Consequences of changing abortion laws, 7-9, 16-17
Constitutional attacks on present abortion laws, 43, 45, 55
Contraceptive measures, 11, 17, 18, 170
Controversial responses to abortion, 173
Costs of abortion, 16, 32
Czechoslovakia, abortion in, 166, 169, 170

Decisions of doctors on abortion, 4, 142-150
Discrimination against poor, 44, 155
Discussion of GAP report, 21-35
District of Columbia abortion decision, 21, 25, 43, 44, 55, 167

Dogmas needing research scrutiny, 10-18

East Germany, abortion in, 17
Educational status of women, 101, 112
Expense to society of abortion, 15

Fetal indication for abortion, 6, 88, 92-97
Finland, abortion in, 111

Great Britain, abortion in, 7, 8, 69-71, 126-130, 168
Griswold decision on abortion, 33, 36, 44
Guilt after abortion, 6, 12, 21, 24, 29-30, 81
Gynecologists concerned with abortion, 26, 65-72, 177-179

Hawaii, abortion in, 46, 162
History of U. S. abortion laws, 54-56
Hungary, abortion in, 110, 120, 166, 169, 170

Illegal effects of abortion, 11, 17, 113-114, 128
Incest and abortion, 86-87
Increased demand for abortion, 126-128, 170
Indications for abortion, 85-88

Japan, abortion in, 8, 11, 15, 26, 32, 33, 110, 120, 168, 169
Justifications for abortion, 42, 69, 167

Legal aspects of abortion, 2-3, 36-47, 167-169
Legal rights of child, 21-35

Marital status of patients, 18, 22, 24, 41, 144, 156
Maryland, abortion in, 24, 162

Massachusetts abortion laws, 41, 51
Medical facilities and manpower for
    abortion, 15-16
Men affected by abortion, 18
Mentally retarded women and abortion, 87
Mortality from abortion, 11, 41, 54, 165-166,
    176-177
Motivations for abortion, 30-31

Negro position on abortion, 32
New Jersey abortion laws, 39, 45
New York City, abortion in, 172-174
New York State, abortion in, 174-175
New York State abortion laws, 36, 39, 46,
    55, 65, 172-173
New York State, guidelines for abortion,
    174-175
Norway, abortion in, 111
Nursing staff attitudes toward abortion,
    59-60

Occupations of husbands, 110

Pennsylvania abortion laws, 43, 65, 67
Personality factors in abortion, 131-141
Peru, abortion in, 15
Policy behind current abortion laws, 37-46
Population problems and abortion, 13-14
Postabortion care and outcome, 160-161
Prediction of disturbances after abortion, 14
Problems of fathers and abortion, 22-23
Psychiatric disorders after abortion, 6, 8-9,
    12, 29-30, 82
Psychiatric indications for abortion, 14-15,
    55-56, 67-69, 73-89, 112-113

Racial factors in abortion, 18, 32, 98-107
Recipients of abortion, 5-6
Refusal of requests for abortion, 12-13,
    57-62, 76-77, 118-119
Religious aspects of abortion, 3, 25, 48-52,
    105-106, 157
Responses to abortion, 80-85
Rights of state, 34, 44-45
Romania, abortion in, 168, 169, 170
Russia, abortion in, 168, 169, 170

Schizophrenia after abortion, 82
Scientific studies of abortion, 74-75
Sexual activity and abortion, 17
Societal attitudes toward abortion, 17
Socioeconomic aspects of abortion, 18,
    108-123
Sterilization as condition for abortion, 76,
    82, 121
Suicidal threats and abortion, 68, 78-80, 85
Swedish studies of abortion, 12, 13, 75,
    80, 116

Therapeutic Abortion Committees, 66-67
Time limits for abortion, 61, 158

United States studies on abortion, 37-46,
    54-56, 112-116, 167-169
Unwanted conceptions, 6-7, 13, 57-62,
    75-78, 119, 130

Vagueness of language in laws on abortion,
    43-44, 55

Wisconsin abortion laws, 55